Get Through

MRCP Part 2: Radiology

Gurmit Singh
Staff Grade in General Medicine and Gastroenterology
Calderdale Royal Hospital
Halifax, West Yorkshire

Hugh Montgomery
Consultant Radiologist
Calderdale Royal Hospital
Halifax, West Yorkshire

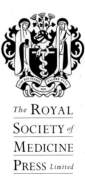

The ROYAL
SOCIETY *of*
MEDICINE
PRESS *Limited*

© 2007 Royal Society of Medicine Press Ltd

Published by the Royal Society of Medicine Press Ltd
1 Wimpole Street, London W1G 0AE, UK
Tel: +44 (0)20 7290 2921
Fax: +44 (0)20 7290 2929
Email: publishing@rsm.ac.uk
Website: www.rsmpress.co.uk

British Library Cataloguing in Publication Data
A catalogue record for this book is available from the British Library

ISBN 978-1-85315-701-1

Distribution in Europe and Rest of World:
Marston Book Services Ltd
PO Box 269
Abingdon
Oxon OX14 4YN, UK
Tel: +44 (0)1235 465500
Fax: +44 (0)1235 465555
Email: direct.order@marston.co.uk

Distribution in the USA and Canada:
Royal Society of Medicine Press Ltd
c/o BookMasters Inc
30 Amberwood Parkway
Ashland, OH 44805, USA
Tel: +1 800 247 6553/+1 800 266 5564
Fax: +1 419 281 6883
Email: order@bookmasters.com

Distribution in Australia and New Zealand:
Elsevier Australia
30–52 Smidmore Street
Marrickville NSW 2204, Australia
Tel: +61 2 9349 5811
Fax: +61 2 9349 5911
Email: service@elsevier.com.au

Phototypeset by Phoenix Photosetting, Chatham, Kent
Printed and bound by Krips b.v., Meppel, The Netherlands

Contents

Foreword

Radiology is a subject that historically has not been given a great deal of exposure at medical school. Much recognition of the patterns of abnormality in differential diagnoses comes to physicians more by osmosis than by much in the way of formal teaching. This book, with its layout of questions related to images, followed by a discussion of the answer and potential differential diagnoses fills a useful role in education. This is not only an examination friendly format but is also a help in the practical assessment of patients and potential differential diagnoses. The question and answer format is laid out so that it can be done either in small chunks or over longer periods of study and should be enjoyable, as well as educational.

No book of this size could ever be comprehensive, but it does cover all the main areas that one would expect, and will be very useful as a revision guide for the MRCP. It also has the benefit that this type of question and answer is quite fun to do, so I can recommend it as a revision aid.

R J H Robertson
Consultant Chest Radiologist &
RCR Regional Education Advisor (Yorkshire)

Preface

This book is intended for candidates preparing for postgraduate medical examinations such as the MRCP, but should also be helpful for medical students and doctors in training. The pattern of the MRCP examination has changed significantly and candidates are now expected not only to identify the features evident in the radiological image shown, but also to formulate a differential diagnosis and know aspects of the necessary management. The scenarios given in the examination are the conditions usually encountered in day-to-day practice, plus some uncommon but 'not to be missed' pathologies.

Radiology has always played a central role in patient management. Candidates going for higher exams are expected to recognize various disease patterns and correlate them with the clinical information provided. We have tried to include the conditions commonly seen in the MRCP exams, and as there is so much to be covered in the huge syllabus, we have included full discussion of the answers as well as background information on certain disease conditions so as to aid the testing and revising process.

This book is a combined effort by a recent MRCP candidate and a consultant radiologist. We would be grateful for any helpful suggestions or constructive criticism to further improve the quality of the book.

Gurmit Singh and Hugh Montgomery

Further reading

Braunwald E et al 2005 Harrison's Principles of Internal Medicine, 16th edn. New York: The McGraw-Hill Companies.

Grainger R, Allison D, Dixon A 2001 Grainger & Allison's Diagnostic Radiology: A textbook of medical imaging, 4th edn. Edinburgh: Churchill Livingstone.

Sutton S 2003 Sutton's Textbook of Radiology and Imaging, 7th edn. Edinburgh: Elsevier Science Ltd.

Warrell DA, Cox TM, Firth JD, Benz EJ, Weatherall D 2005 Oxford Textbook of Medicine, 4th edn. Oxford: Oxford University Press.

www.emedicine.com

www.montymedia.net – an expanding archive of interactive material with an emphasis on image interpretation.

Dedicated to my wife, Manpreet, and
my lovely son, Savi

Gurmit

Acknowledgements

I am extremely thankful to my co-author, Dr Hugh Montgomery; without his support this book would not have been possible. Dr Montgomery is a consultant radiologist at Calderdale Royal Hospital, Halifax and his main interests are ultrasound, CT and interventional radiology. He takes great interest in teaching. He has also produced a website aimed mainly at junior doctors that has quality teaching material available (www.montymedia.net).

I am very grateful to Dr Steve Thomas, who has been very supportive, and for reading and commenting on the text. I would also like to thank Dr Rod Robertson (Consultant Radiologist, Leeds General Infirmary) for his valuable suggestions and support. I am also thankful to Dr Brian Lalor for his constant encouragement and infusing in me the passion for clinical medicine.

This book would have been impossible without the support of my wife and I am indebted to her and my 6-year-old son for the patience they have shown while I was working on it.

I am also very grateful to my friends Prabal, Dr Deepashree and Dr Thomas's secretary, Barbara for their help.

Gurmit

Section 1: Chest

Questions

1.1 A 45-year-old man presented with complaints of malaise, fever, cough and mucopurulent nasal discharge of 3 months' duration. Blood tests revealed mild anaemia, elevated white cell count (WCC), CRP 120 and renal impairment. A recent chest X-ray (top) and a previous X-ray (bottom) are shown. What is the most likely diagnosis?

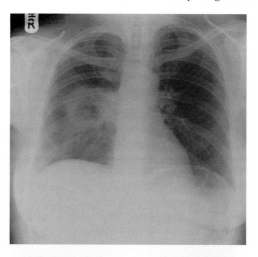

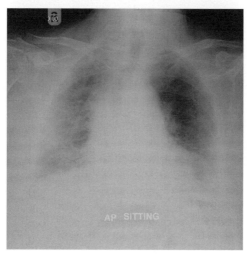

A. Tuberculosis
B. Polyarteritis nodosa
C. Histoplasmosis
D. Wegener's granulomatosis

1.2 All the following are features of the above diagnosis except:

A. Upper respiratory disease
B. Lower respiratory disease
C. Glomerulonephritis
D. Asthma

1.3 Choose the correct option in relation to the above diagnosis:

A. Radiologically, presence of cavitation is considered to be characteristic.
B. Hypogammaglobulinemia
C. p-ANCA
D. The nodules on chest X-ray persist even after treatment.

1.4 A 55-year-old man had presented with complaints of weight loss, malaise, cough and shortness of breath. Blood tests revealed raised white cell count (WCC) and also showed high lactose dehydrogenase (LDH) levels. The images are shown. What is the most likely diagnosis?

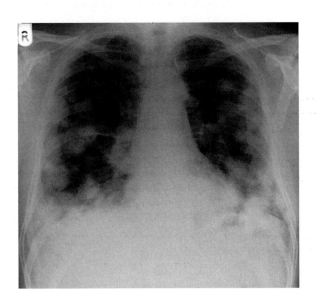

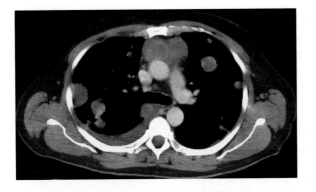

A. Histoplasmosis
B. Wegener's granulomatosis
C. Mediastinal germ cell tumour with lung metastases
D. Staphylococcal abscesses

1.5 What other tests are required to aid diagnosis?

A. CEA
B. CA 199
C. AST
D. AFP and B-HCG

1.6 Choose the correct response:

A. Retroperitoneum is the most common site of extragonadal primary germ cell tumour.
B. Elevation of AFP is higher than B-HCG in mediastinal non-seminomatous germ cell tumour.
C. The tumour markers AFP and B-HCG do not provide prognostic information.
D. A testicular ultrasound should be arranged in all cases with mediastinal non-seminomatous germ cell tumour.

1.7 A 32-year-old man presented with cough, dyspnoea, redness of the eyes and joint pains. Initial blood tests showed a raised erythrocyte sedimentation rate (ESR), low lymphocyte count and eosinophilia. A CXR and CT scan were done and are shown. What is the likely diagnosis?

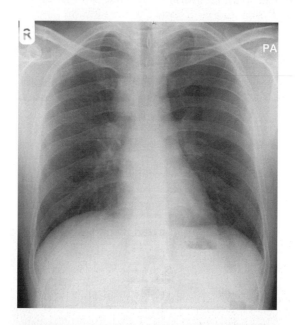

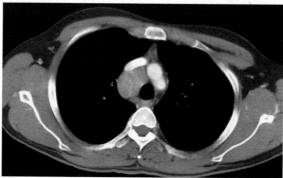

A. Tuberculosis
B. Lymphoma
C. Sarcoidosis
D. Brucellosis

1.8 Regarding the chest X-ray findings in sarcoidosis choose the correct answer:

A. The CXR is abnormal at some stage in only 50% of cases.
B. Egg shell calcification of the lymph nodes may be seen.
C. Parenchymal opacities usually involve the lower lobes.
D. Pleural effusion is never a feature of sarcoidosis.

1.9 All the following are true of sarcoidosis except:

A. Skin anergy is seen in sarcoidosis.
B. Elevated 24-hour urinary calcium.
C. The ACE levels may be indicative of disease activity.
D. Pneumothorax is very commonly associated with sarcoidosis.

1.10 This chest X-ray was carried out on a routine basis on an asymptomatic 50-year-old man with no previous significant medical history. What is the diagnosis?

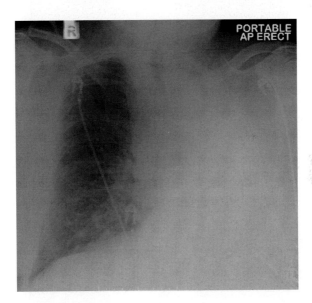

A. Massive pleural effusion
B. Lung collapse
C. Lung hypoplasia
D. Consolidation

1.11 All the following are true of pulmonary agenesis except:

A. The mediastinum is shifted towards affected side.
B. Due to interruption in the vascular supply to the lung bud during foetal development.
C. The main bronchus and lung are absent on the affected side.
D. On angiography the pulmonary artery is seen on affected side.

1.12 A 58-year-old woman presented with difficulty in swallowing and neck fullness. A chest X-ray and CT were carried out and the images are shown. On further examination she was found to be having facial congestion, engorged neck veins and she almost fainted when her arms were raised above her head. The name of this clinical sign is:

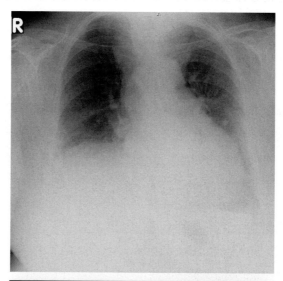

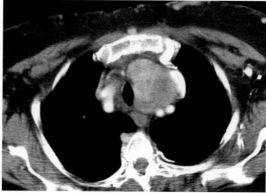

A. Pemburton's sign
B. Hamman's sign
C. Lhermitte's sign
D. Murphy's sign

1.13 All the following tumours are commonly seen in anterior mediastinum, except:

A. Thymic tumours
B. Germ cell tumour
C. Thyroid mass
D. Neurogenic tumours

1.14 All the following are true regarding a mediastinal mass except:

A. For further evaluation CT scan and lung function tests are helpful.
B. Thymus is abnormal in 75% of patients with myasthenia gravis.
C. Teratoma has an association with thymic enlargement.
D. Only 25% of patients with myasthenia gravis show improvement in their symptoms after thymectomy.

1.15 A 55-year-old man presented with chest discomfort and haemoptysis. His past medical history consists of tuberculosis, which was treated, and ulcerative colitis, for which he is on azathioprine. A chest X-ray was carried out and is shown. What is the most likely pathology?

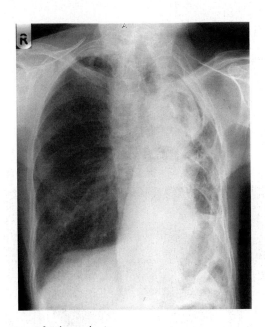

A. Reactivation of tuberculosis
B. Aspergilloma
C. Bronchogenic cyst
D. Lung carcinoma

1.16 Choose the correct response:

    A. Aspergilloma should be treated with intravenous amphotericin even if asymptomatic.

    B. The fungal ball seen on CXR should move when the patient position is changed.

    C. Bronchial artery embolization is preferred to surgical resection of the affected lobe, even in fit patients.

    D. Aspergilloma is most commonly seen in the lower zone of lung.

1.17 A 52-year-old man presented with vomiting and later developed chest pain, breathlessness and fever. An initial chest X-ray was normal but the chest X-ray repeated on the next day is shown along with the CT scan. What is the diagnosis?

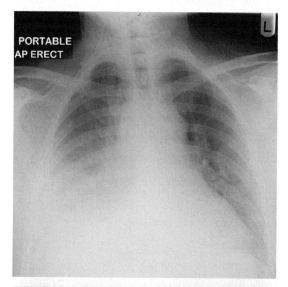

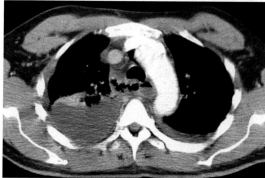

    A. Rupture of the oesophagus

    B. Pneumonia

    C. Acute pancreatitis

    D. Rupture of the intra-abdominal viscus

1.18 All the following are true except:

    A. Hamman's sign may be present in cases of pneumomediastinum.
    B. Salivary amylase in pleural fluid is elevated in oesophageal rupture.
    C. Boerhaave's syndrome is traumatic rupture of the oesophagus.
    D. Treatment of oesophageal rupture involves broad-spectrum antibiotics and urgent surgical repair.

1.19 A 68-year-old man who has worked as a pipe fitter all his life presented with breathlessness on exertion and chest discomfort. A chest X-ray was carried out and is shown along with the CT scan. What do you think is the diagnosis?

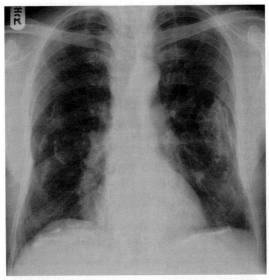

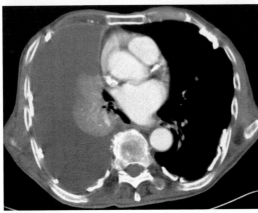

    A. Tuberculosis
    B. Asbestosis
    C. Sarcoidosis
    D. Carcinoma of the lung

1.20 All the following are true except:

    A. Presence of pleural plaque is indicative of previous exposure to asbestos.

    B. The risk of developing cancer increases significantly with smoking.

    C. Peritoneal mesothelioma is not associated with asbestos exposure.

    D. The opacities on CXR seen with asbestosis are first seen in the lower zones.

1.21 A 40-year-old man had a routine chest X-ray (shown). What is the diagnosis?

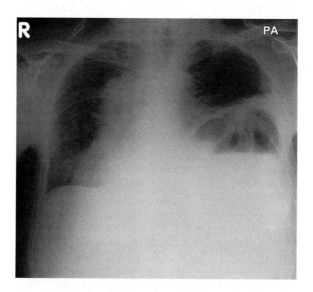

    A. Eventration of the diaphragm

    B. Hiatus hernia

    C. Bochdalek's hernia

    D. Morgagni hernia

1.22 All the following are true regarding traumatic rupture of the diaphragm except:

    A. The mediastinum shifts towards the contralateral side.

    B. The mediastinum shifts towards the ipsilateral side.

    C. The NG tube may be seen in the hemithorax.

    D. The bowel loops may not be visible in the abdomen.

1.23 In the images shown, what is the most likely diagnosis?

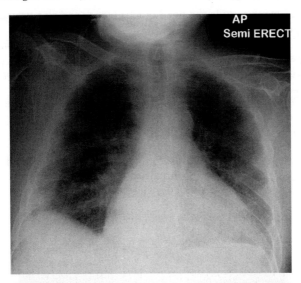

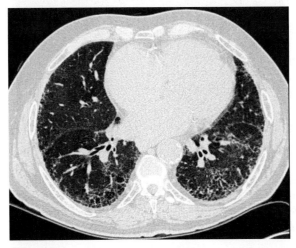

A. Coal worker's pneumoconiosis
B. Lung involvement in ankylosing spondylitis
C. CFA
D. Histiocytosis X

1.24 The patient complains of sudden worsening of dyspnoea with associated chest pain, what complication might have occurred?

A. Infection
B. Pulmonary embolism
C. Pneumothorax
D. Anxiety

1.25 Select most appropriate response:

    A. HRCT may preclude the need of lung biopsy and also provide information on prognosis in CFA.

    B. HRCT appearance of sarcoidosis may show a predilection for the lung bases.

    C. Pleural effusion in rheumatoid lung disease is more common in men than in women.

    D. DTPA scanning should be done routinely in assessment of interstitial lung diseases.

1.26 A 45-year-old woman who is a known alcoholic presented with cough, a copious amount of sputum production and chest discomfort. The images are shown. What is your diagnosis?

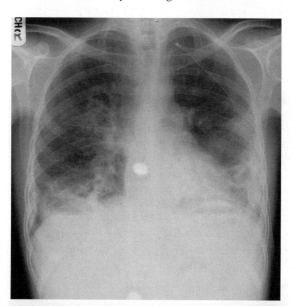

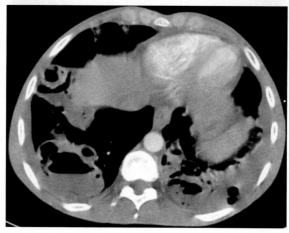

A. Pulmonary cyst
B. Aspergilloma
C. Lung abscess
D. Hydatid cyst

1.27 All the following are true except:

   A. A nodular margin of the abscess cavity may be seen in squamous cell carcinoma.
   B. Multiple cavities may be seen in the case of metastatic lung abscess.
   C. On CT scan the abscess wall makes an acute angle with the chest wall.
   D. An antibiotic course for 2 weeks clears the infection in most cases.

1.28 A 62-year-old man who is a heavy smoker presented with cough, breathlessness and weight loss. He was found to have finger clubbing. A chest X-ray was arranged and is shown. What is the most likely diagnosis?

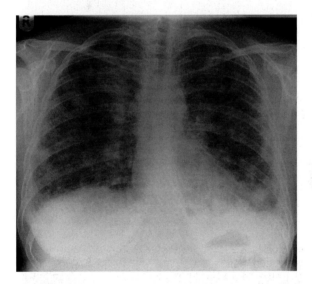

   A. Histoplasmosis
   B. Wegener's granulomatosis
   C. Lung metastases
   D. Sarcoidosis

1.29 Abscopal effect (spontaneous resolution of lung secondaries when primary is treated) is seen with:

   A. Colonic cancer
   B. Trophoblastic tumours
   C. Hepatocellular carcinoma
   D. Malignant melanoma

1.30 All are true regarding pulmonary metastases except:

    A. Cavitation is commonly seen with metastatic adenocarcinoma.

    B. Metastatic squamous cell carcinoma has a predilection for upper lobes.

    C. The usual distribution of lung metastases is in the peripheral or basal region.

    D. Calcification is an uncommon feature of lung metastases.

1.31 A 42-year-old man who was previously fit and well presented with mild cough and chills of 1-week duration. The blood tests revealed high white cell count and a C-reactive protein (CRP) of 110. A chest X-ray was carried out and is shown. What is the most likely cause?

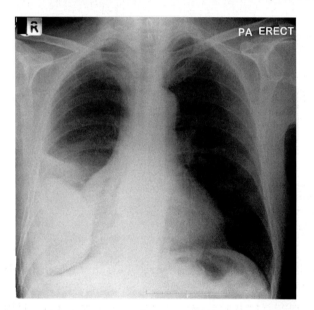

    A. Tuberculosis

    B. Round pneumonia

    C. Carcinoma of the lung

    D. Aspergilloma

1.32 All of the following are true regarding round pneumonia except:

    A. It is more common in children.

    B. It usually involves the lower lobe of the lung.

    C. A course of antibiotics leads to complete resolution of the opacity.

    D. Air bronchograms are characteristic of round pneumonia and are helpful to differentiate it from carcinoma.

1.33 A 40-year-old man presented with a history of dry cough, breathlessness on exertion and fever. He was hypoxemic and blood tests showed mild leucocytosis and elevated lactose dehydrogenase (LDH) levels. A chest X-ray was carried out. What do you think is the diagnosis?

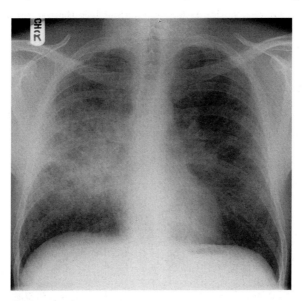

    A. Tuberculosis
    B. Pulmonary oedema
    C. *Pneumocystis carinii* pneumonia (PCP)
    D. Cryptogenic organizing pneumonia

1.34 Regarding aerosolized pentamidine used in PCP prophylaxis, please choose the best response:

    A. Pneumothorax is a recognized complication and can be difficult to treat.
    B. Pneumothorax always resolves with intercostal tube drainage.
    C. It is more effective than co-trimoxazole.
    D. On chest X-ray, lower lobe infiltrates are seen when PCP occurs during aerosolized pentamidine therapy.

1.35 Choose the best response:

    A. Pleural effusion and lymphadenopathy are common radiographic features of PCP.
    B. Spontaneous pneumothorax, a known complication of PCP, is always unilateral.
    C. PCP is unlikely in the presence of normal TLCO and normal HRCT.
    D. A CXR is always abnormal in PCP.

1.36 A 46-year-old woman who is known to have severe rheumatoid arthritis presented with a dry cough and breathlessness, both at rest and on exertion and mild fever. Blood tests showed slightly raised white cell count and eosinophil count. The images are shown. Choose the correct option:

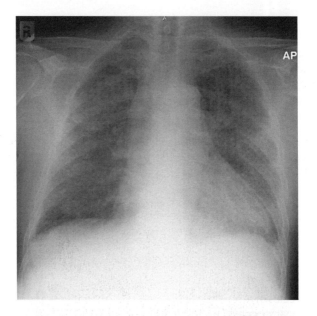

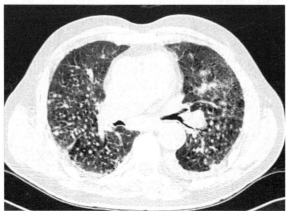

A. Diffuse pulmonary lung disease associated with rheumatoid arthritis
B. Tuberculosis
C. Drug-induced lung disease secondary to methotrexate
D. *Pneumocystis carinii* pneumonia

1.37 Regarding drug-induced lung disease, the following is correct:

A. Pleural effusion is common.
B. In systemic lupus-like syndrome caused by drugs, kidneys are not involved.
C. Lymphadenopathy is a prominent feature.
D. Upper lung zones are mainly affected.

1.38 Hilar lymphadenopathy can be seen with:

A. Salicylates
B. Bleomycin
C. Phenytoin
D. Gold

1.39 A 20-year-old man who is tall and thin presented with chest pain and shortness of breath. A chest X-ray was carried out and is shown. It is likely that the patient has:

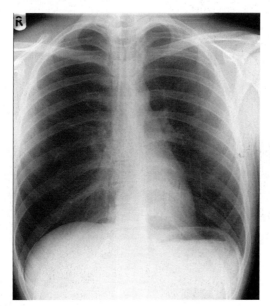

A. Klinefelter's syndrome
B. Marfan's syndrome
C. Kalman's syndrome
D. Addison's disease

1.40 Regarding catamenial pneumothorax, all the following are true except:

A. Always associated with endometriosis
B. Most common in parous women in fourth decade of life
C. Commonly occurs on the right side
D. Can be recurrent

1.41 Choose the correct response:

A. Pneumothorax in PCP resolves quickly with intercostal tube drainage.
B. A CT scan is a more sensitive investigation in suspected pneumothorax than a chest X-ray.
C. A patient with SSP who was minimally breathless and with a small pneumothorax (size < 1 cm) can be safely discharged after aspiration.
D. Pneumothorax is very rare in lymphangioleiomyomatosis.

Answers

1.1   D
1.2   D
1.3   A

Wegener's granulomatosis

Wegener's granulomatosis is a vasculitic disorder characterized by the triad of upper and lower respiratory disease and glomerulonephritis. The cause is unknown but immunological mechanisms are thought to be responsible. The pathological hallmark is necrotizing vasculitis of small arteries and veins together with granuloma formation, which may be intravascular or extravascular.

Clinical features
Onset may be acute or insidious. Signs and symptoms consist of fever, weight loss, rash, rhinitis, otitis, nasal congestion and discharge, cough, dyspnoea and haemoptysis. Other features include polyarthritis which may be migratory, episcleritis, conjunctivitis, proptosis and epistaxis. Coronary artery involvement may lead to MI and renovascular hypertension may be present.

Investigations
The condition should be suspected if there are unexplained and ongoing upper or lower respiratory symptoms, particularly in the presence of renal involvement. Blood tests may show anaemia, mild leukocytosis, high ESR, thrombocytosis, hypergammaglobinaemia and presence of rheumatoid factor. Serum ANCA helps in diagnosis. It is highly specific but not diagnostic. The cytoplasmic pattern caused by antibodies to proteinase 3, which is a constituent of neutrophil granules, has a specificity of > 90% for Wegener's granulomatosis.

   A CXR should be obtained first followed by a CT scan of the chest. In the presence of symptoms CT scan of the paranasal sinuses may be needed. The diagnosis is further confirmed by tissue biopsy, which will reveal necrotizing granulomatous vasculitis. Pulmonary tissue has the highest yield.

Radiology
CXR may show multiple nodular shadows or masses. It may also be seen as a solitary pulmonary nodule. A CT of the chest is helpful in defining the extent of the pulmonary involvement. Presence of a cavitating lesion(s) is considered to be characteristic of Wegener's but may not be always present. Multiple nodules and areas of consolidation representing haemorrhage may be present.

Differential diagnosis
* Tuberculosis
* Lung abscess

- Carcinoma of the lung
- Aspergilloma
- Histoplasmosis

Treatment
It is invariably fatal if left untreated. Early treatment is crucial to prevent further progression and renal failure. Most effective therapy is combination of cyclophosphamide and glucocorticoids. With this regime marked improvement is seen in > 90% of patients and in 75% complete remission is seen.

1.4 C
1.5 D
1.6 D

Mediastinal germ cell tumours

The mediastinum is the most common site of extragonadal germ cell tumour (EGGCT). They constitute about 10–15% of all mediastinal neoplasms. They can also be found in other sites like the retroperitoneum. The malignant germ cell tumours (GCTs) can be divided into seminomas and non-seminomatous type. Non-seminomatous GCTs are almost exclusively seen in men and they can be associated with Klinefelter's syndrome.

Clinical features
Mediastinal EGGCT can present with chest pain, cough, dyspnoea, fever, weight loss and anorexia. The most common site in the mediastinum is the anterosuperior compartment and they tend to grow rapidly and metastasize early.

Investigations
Blood tests usually reveal high B-HCG and AFP levels. Elevation of B-HCG is higher in patients with mediastinal non-seminomatous GCT than in those with primary metastatic testicular tumours and can be used as a marker to assess response to treatment and to detect recurrence. Most of the patients have high LDH levels though it is a non-specific marker. These tumour markers provide diagnostic and prognostic information. Histopathology is crucial to diagnosis but if it is not possible because of poor general condition then treatment can be started even without biopsy in the presence of radiological findings and high serum markers.

Radiology
Imaging plays important role in the diagnosis and further management. It helps to identify the mass, define its extent and presence of metastatic disease. A CXR may show enlargement of the mediastinum and the tumour may appear lobular in outline. It may also reveal lung metastases.

The CT scan is the imaging modality of choice. In all patients CT of the thorax, abdomen and pelvis should be performed. The mediastinal non-seminomatous GCT may be seen as a large, irregular mass situated in the anterior mediastinum. The CT also shows metastases to the lung, liver, lymph nodes and bones. A testicular ultrasound should be arranged in all cases with an extragonadal GCT.

Treatment and prognosis

The mainstay of treatment is chemotherapy. The patients may require postchemotherapy surgical resection. With cisplatin-based chemotherapy the prognosis may range between 50 and 70%. Prognosis is said to be poorer with primary mediastinal non-seminomatous GCT.

1.7 C
1.8 D
1.9 D

Sarcoidosis

Sarcoidosis is a chronic multisystem granulomatous disease of unknown aetiology. Most patients present between 20 and 40 years. It is more commonly seen in people of Afro-Caribbean origin. It may be discovered incidentally during a CXR performed routinely.

Clinical features

It is a disease of young adults but may be seen in all age groups and it may present insidiously over a period of months. It may present acutely with erythema nodosum and polyarthritis. Chest symptoms include cough, dyspnoea, and chest pain. Extrapulmonary manifestations may include uveitis, parotid enlargement, hepatomegaly, splenomegaly, neuropathy, lupus pernio, subcutaneous nodules, arrhythmias and meningitis.

In the acute form, two syndromes are described:

- Lofgren's syndrome is the presence of erythema nodosum, arthritis and bilateral hilar lymphadenopathy.
- Heerfordt-Waldenstrom syndrome is characterized by the presence of uveitis, fever, enlarged parotid glands and facial nerve palsy.

Diagnosis

Diagnosis is by a combination of clinical, radiological and pathological findings. Blood tests may show high ESR, lymphopenia, eosinophilia, raised serum immunoglobulins, calcium and ACE levels. Other investigations like CT scan of the chest and abdomen, lung function tests and bronchoscopy may be required. Tissue biopsy is usually diagnostic. Bronchoalveolar lavage may show increased lymphocytes. Definite diagnosis is by a tissue biopsy. Slit lamp examination is indicated in ocular disease.

Radiology

CXR is abnormal at some stage in 90% of cases. Three classic patterns of CXR findings are:

Type 1: Bilateral hilar lymphadenopathy (BHL) with no parenchymal abnormalities
Type 2: BHL with diffuse parenchymal changes
Type 3: Diffuse parenchymal changes without BHL

The BHL is usually symmetrical and if it is not, other diagnoses should be considered. Other CXR findings include eggshell calcification of the hilar nodes, pleural effusion, cavity formation and fibrosis. Parenchymal opacities usually show mid- and upper zone involvement.

Other causes for BHL:

- Lymphoma
- Tuberculosis
- Neoplasia
- Brucellosis

Other causes for eggshell calcification of lymph nodes:

- Histoplasmosis
- Silicosis
- Post-irradiation lymphoma

Gallium-67 scan is abnormal showing diffuse uptake but is not diagnostic. CT/MRI may be helpful in assessing severity and in neurosarcoidosis.

Treatment and prognosis
The mainstay of treatment is glucocorticoids. They are not indicated in BHL alone in asymptomatic individuals. Prognosis is generally good.

1.10 C
1.11 D

Opaque hemithorax

When complete opacification of hemithorax is seen on a CXR it should be interpreted in the context of clinical presentation. In some cases the condition may be present from birth. It is of utmost importance to look for mediastinal shift (position of trachea and heart).

Causes
It may be encountered in the following conditions:

- *Large pleural effusion*: the mediastinum may shift away from the affected side. If there is no mediastinal shift, underlying collapse of the lung should be considered.
- *Consolidation*: as seen in severe pneumonia. There is usually no mediastinal shift.
- *Post pneumonectomy*: the mediastinum shifts towards affected side.
- *Lung collapse*: the mediastinum is shifted towards the affected side. The causes may be extrinsic or intrinsic. Some common causes include: lymph nodes and masses outside the bronchus, mucoid impaction, an inhaled foreign body, tuberculosis, sarcoidosis, lung cancer etc.

Pulmonary agenesis
It is a rare cause of opaque hemithorax. It is usually due to interruption in the vascular supply to the lung bud during foetal development. On the CXR the mediastinum may be shifted towards the affected side. The other lung may appear hyperexpanded. The CT scan shows absence of the main

bronchus and lung on the affected side. Angiography shows absence of the pulmonary artery on that side.

1.12 A
1.13 D
1.14 D

Mediastinal mass

The mediastinum can be divided into three compartments: anterior, middle and posterior. Masses arising from one compartment may cross to another. If a mediastinal mass is seen in the frontal film, a lateral film should be obtained. Further evaluation with CT is required.

Causes

- *Anterior mediastinum*: thyroid masses, thymic tumours, germ cell tumour or teratoma
- *Middle mediastinum*: vascular anamolies, bronchogenic cyst, lymphadenopathy due to tuberculosis, histoplasmosis, sarcoidosis, metastasis and lymphoma
- *Posterior mediastinum*: neurofibroma, neurogenic tumours, spinal tumours

Thyroid mass
Intrathoracic thyroid shows round or lobular outline. Retrosternal goitre may obstruct the thoracic inlet. It can also compress the large airways. Pemburton's sign may be positive (facial congestion and faintness when arms are raised above the head). Further evaluation should be carried out with lung function studies and CT/MRI.

Thymic tumours
They may be benign or malignant. They are frequently associated with myasthenia gravis. The thymus is abnormal in about 75% cases of myasthenia and about 85% of patients feel improvement after thymectomy. Many other conditions may be associated with thymic enlargement including teratoma, hypogammaglobulinaemia and Cushing's disease.

Teratoma/germ cell tumour (GCT)
Teratomas are more commonly seen than GCT. They may be diagnosed incidentally on a routine CXR or secondary to local symptoms like cough or chest pain. A CT is helpful for further evaluation. It may show calcification or a cystic mass. A malignant GCT secretes B-HCG and AFP. They are fast growing and metastasize early. A CXR may show a lobular mediastinal mass. A CT is required for further evaluation (see also section 1.2)

1.15 B
1.16 B

Aspergilloma

Aspergillosis is an opportunistic infection caused by *Aspergillus* sp. It is one of the most commonly found environmental moulds. It is usually inhaled but can also invade broken/denuded skin. It may be locally invasive and may lead to disseminated infection in susceptible individuals.

Aspergilloma (fungal ball) is a tangled mass of *Aspergillus* hyphae. It is a non-invasive or minimally invasive form and occurs secondary to colonization of pulmonary cavities like old tuberculosis, lung cancer and bronchiectasis. Invasive aspergillosis may ensue in susceptible individuals.

Risk factors
Neutropenia, immunosuppression, e.g. in long-term corticosteroid therapy, post-transplant patients and AIDS.

Clinical features
Aspergilloma may be asymptomatic. It may cause some chest discomfort. In invasive types systemic symptoms, cough and wheezing may occur. Occasionally it can lead to haemoptysis, which may be life threatening.

Diagnosis
Serum IgE concentrations may be elevated. IgG antibody to *Aspergillus* antigen is usually demonstrable. Sputum culture is not usually helpful.

Radiology
X-ray may show a fungal ball within a cavity that may move with change of position. The crescent sign may be seen, which is a crescent-shaped air space separating the fungal ball from the cavity wall. CT scanning is usually required for further evaluation. The crescent of air may be better seen on CT than on a plain film. Pleural thickening may be seen.

Differential diagnosis
- Tuberculosis
- Neoplasia
- Lung abscess
- Wegener's granulomatosis
- Bronchogenic cyst

Treatment
Asymptomatic aspergillomas do not need treatment. However, complications like haemoptysis may occur, which may necessitate lobectomy. In some cases bronchial artery embolization may help. Antifungal treatment is not helpful in the treatment of the fungal ball. Intravenous amphotericin may be required if there is evidence of invasive aspergillosis. Liposomal amphotericin may be preferable due to lesser side effects.

1.17 A
1.18 C

Oesophageal rupture

Rupture of the oesophagus is an emergency. If urgent repair of the perforation is not carried out it has a high mortality rate.

Causes

- Iatrogenic – during instrumentation of the oesophagus and dilatation
- Spontaneous rupture – also called Boerhaave's syndrome. This is usually secondary to retching or vomiting.
- Trauma
- Oesophageal diseases like ulcer or neoplasia

Clinical features

There may be a history of recent instrumentation or the patient may be having retching and vomiting. The patient may complain of chest or abdominal pain, cough, dyspnoea, haematemesis or features of shock. In the elderly and patients taking steroids the presentation may not be dramatic.

Subcutaneous emphysema may be palpable in the neck and over the chest wall. Pneumothorax or pneumomediastinum may occur. Eventually secondary infection supervenes. On auscultation a crunching sound synchronous with each heart beat may be heard (Hamman's sign) when there is air in the mediastinum.

Differential diagnosis

- Acute pancreatitis
- Myocardial infarction
- Acute cholecystitis
- Pneumonia
- Rupture of intra-abdominal viscus

Diagnosis

Blood tests show raised inflammatory markers. Pleural fluid has a high salivary amylase content.

Radiology

Imaging plays a crucial role to aid diagnosis. A CXR should be carried out urgently and it may show pleural effusion, mediastinal air or pneumothorax. It may also show surgical emphysema. CT gives more detailed information and may reveal small leakage of air in the mediastinum but it may fail to show the site of leakage. Contrast study with a non-ionic water-soluble contrast agent usually reveals the site of rupture.

Treatment

Keep nil by mouth, with circulatory support, broad-spectrum antibiotics and urgent surgical repair.

1.19 B
1.20 C

Asbestos-related disorders

Asbestos-related disorders are caused by inhalation of asbestos fibres. This usually occurs at the workplace as seen in workers involved in mining and manufacturing, construction, shipbuilding, pipe fitters and boilermakers. Exposure may also occur in people not directly exposed to asbestos, for example the wife of a shipbuilder who washes her husband's clothes.

The spectrum of conditions may range from pleural thickening, pleural plaques, benign pleural effusions, asbestosis, lung cancer (non-small cell) and mesothelioma. The risk of lung cancer is 8–10 times more than in people not exposed to asbestos. Smoking further increases the risk.

Asbestosis

It is a form of diffuse interstitial lung disease. Severity of the condition depends on duration and intensity of exposure but also depends on the type of asbestos fibre. In about 10% of people the condition may progress even after cessation of exposure. It may be aysmptomatic initially and later on causes malaise, breathlessness and a dry cough. In severe cases features of right heart failure may be present.

To establish the diagnosis a history of exposure should be sought. Lung function studies may reveal a restrictive pattern, reduced lung volumes and with reduction of TLCO. Imaging plays a crucial role in diagnosis. Bronchoalveolar lavage may be helpful and lung biopsy is seldom required.

Radiology

The CXR features may be similar to those of fibrosing alveolitis and may be difficult to distinguish. It may show irregular or linear opacities seen peripherally in lung bases and later it may spread to the middle and upper zones with associated pleural changes. The diaphragm and heart border (shaggy heart sign) may appear indistinct. HRCT is particularly helpful for further evaluation. Parenchymal fibrotic bands and subpleural curvilinear lines that appear parallel to the pleural surface may be seen. Both an HRCT and standard-resolution CT scan should be obtained.

There is no specific treatment. Pulmonary rehabilitation and preventive measures like stopping exposure, smoking cessation and pneumococcal and influenza vaccination may improve quality of life.

Pleural disease

This is the hallmark of asbestos exposure. Presence of pleural plaques does not necessarily mean lung involvement. On CXR pleural plaques are most commonly seen in the lower lung zones, diaphragm and abutting cardiac border. Pleural effusions are less common. They may appear haemorrhagic and are exudative. They usually resolve spontaneously.

Malignant mesotheliomas may arise from pleural plaques. They may present with chest pain and dyspnoea. Spread to adjacent organs may cause hoarseness of voice, Horner's syndrome and dysphagia.

Radiology

CXR may show unilateral or bilateral pleural thickening. There may be blunting of the costophrenic angle and the lung may appear to be encased within the thickening. Pleural effusions, which may be massive, may be seen. A staging CT should be arranged, which is used to assess the extent of disease.

Surgery or radiotherapy may be required but they may not improve survival. The prognosis remains poor.

Unilateral elevation of diaphragm

The diaphragm is a thin sheet of muscle with an upward convexity. The changes in height or shape of the diaphragm may give clues to the underlying pathological changes. In 90% of people the right hemidiaphragm lies at a higher level than the left side.

Causes of unilateral elevation of diaphragm

- Lung agenesis/hypoplasia
- Gaseous distension of stomach or colon
- Phrenic nerve palsy – malignancy, neurological conditions
- Eventration of the diaphragm
- Pulmonary embolism
- Pneumonia
- Lung collapse
- Subphrenic mass/abscess
- Traumatic rupture of diaphragm

Clinical features

History plays a very important role. When the rupture is traumatic, along with the history of trauma patients may be having abdominal pain that may radiate towards the ipsilateral shoulder; cardiac dysrhythmias or respiratory distress may be present. Later, there may be chest pain, vomiting or breathlessness.

In diaphragmatic palsy secondary to neurological conditions, some patients may be asymptomatic. There may be breathlessness or they may get breathless when lying on the affected side.

Diagnosis

Lung function tests in both supine and erect positions may be helpful.

Radiology

CXR shows the presence of an elevated diaphragm. It may also show any lesions affecting the phrenic nerve. Fluoroscopy is helpful in further evaluation. Paradoxical movement may be noticed on inspiration in paralysis of the diaphragm. In cases of trauma or congenital hernias, abdominal contents are visible in the chest on the affected side. In traumatic rupture of the diaphragm, the mediastinum may shift to the contralateral side. The bowel loops may not be visible in the abdomen. If an NG tube is passed it may be seen lying in the hemithorax.

MRI is helpful in further evaluation of the diaphragm.

Causes of bilateral elevation of the diaphragm

- Obesity
- Poor inspiratory effort
- Ascites
- Pregnancy

- Diffuse pulmonary fibrosis
- Bilateral diaphragmatic paralysis

Flattening of the diaphragm may be seen in emphysema. Contrary to popular belief, a difference in the levels of both hemidiaphragms is related to the position of the cardiac apex and not to the liver.

1.23 C
1.24 C
1.25 A

Diffuse parenchymal lung disease

Diffuse parenchymal lung disease (DPLD) is becoming the preferred term instead of interstitial lung disease. It consists of a large number of disease conditions that affect the pulmonary interstitium. The spectrum of DPLD is very wide with different aetiological, pathological and prognostic factors. Readers are advised to refer to standard textbooks for a detailed classification. A few causes are mentioned here:

1. *Idiopathic*: cryptogenic fibrosing alveolitis (CFA)
2. *Environmental agents*:
   - Inorganic dusts: asbestos, silicosis, siderosis
   - Organic dusts: farmer's lung (thermoactinomycetes), bird fancier's lung (avian protein allergy)
3. *Connective tissue diseases/vasculitides*: sarcoidosis, ankylosing spondylitis, rheumatoid arthritis, systemic lupus erythematosus, polymyositis, Wegener's granulomatosis
4. *Infections*: tuberculosis (TB), histoplasmosis, opportunistic infections like *pneumocystis carinii* pneumonia (PCP), invasive aspergillosis
5. *Drugs*: amiodarone, methotrexate, bleomycin, gold
6. *Miscellaneous*: radiation pneumonitis, inflammatory bowel disease, lymphoma

Clinical features
The onset can be acute or chronic. Acute presentation is commonly seen with infections like TB, invasive aspergillosis, *Pneumocystis carinii* infection, hypersensitivity pneumonitis or drugs. Otherwise, it follows a chronic course. The most common symptom is dyspnoea. Other symptoms include dry cough, chest pain or discomfort, fatigue and weight loss. Pneumothorax should be suspected in a patient with DPLD with sudden worsening of dyspnoea.

On physical examination, clubbing, cyanosis (usually a late feature) and tachypnoea may be present. On chest auscultation fine end-inspiratory crepitations may be heard over the lobe(s) of the lung involved. It is important to look for associated systemic features. In the late stages of the disease, signs of pulmonary hypertension or cor pulmonale may be present.

Diagnosis

Clinical assessment
A proper history is very important. It should include the mode of onset, associated systemic features, presence of other disease conditions, smoking

and family history, drug history both current and past, occupational history, hobbies and a search for immunosuppressive conditions. This should be followed by a thorough physical examination.

Laboratory tests
These include full blood count including eosinophil count, urea and electrolytes, liver function tests, serum immunoglobulins, ESR, rheumatoid factor, ANCA and serum precipitins. Blood gases shows hypoxemia with low/normal PCO_2.

Radiology
A CXR should be obtained but it may be normal initially. High-resolution CT (HRCT) scan is the imaging modality of choice.

Chest X-ray
There is a poor correlation between a CXR and the clinical condition or the pathological stage. The differential diagnosis can be narrowed with the type of opacity and part of the lung involved. If a CXR is normal, a HRCT should be arranged.

The patterns of radiographic abnormality in DPLD can be reticular, nodular, septal, ground glass and reticulonodular. Some examples of each type are given below:

- *Reticular*: asbestosis, CFA, sarcoidosis, rheumatoid lung disease
- *Nodular*: silicosis, coal worker's pneumoconiosis
- *Septal*: lymphangitis carcinomatosis
- *Ground glass*: extrinsic allergic alveolitis, PCP
- *Reticulonodular*: histiocytosis X, sarcoidosis

Causes of upper zone involvement:

- Ankylosing spondylitis
- Silicosis (may involve mid zone)
- Coal worker's pneumoconiosis (upper and mid zone)
- Tuberculosis
- Histiocytosis X (eosinophilic granuloma)
- Invasive allergic bronchopulmonary aspergillosis (may also involve the lower lobe)

Causes of lower zone involvement:

- Cryptogenic fibrosing alveolitis
- Systemic sclerosis/polymyositis
- Asbestosis
- Rheumatoid arthritis
- Drugs and radiation

HRCT
This is a very sensitive imaging modality and is useful when a CXR is normal. The distribution and type of the parenchymal disease, for example interstitial, ground-glass opacities or honeycombing can provide valuable

information on the type of DPLD, which can sometimes preclude the need for a biopsy. It can provide prognostic information in CFA. It can also help to identify an appropriate biopsy site.

Pulmonary function tests

A restrictive defect is seen and also a reduced gas transfer factor. Sometimes an obstructive pattern may be seen with some DPLDs and hence a finding of airflow obstruction does not rule out the presence of DPLD. Vital capacity and gas transfer factor are helpful in disease monitoring.

Bronchoscopy and bronchoalveolar lavage (BAL)

BAL may provide diagnostic and prognostic information. It can be useful in diagnosis of opportunistic infections, malignancy, occupational, drug-induced and granulomatous DPLDs. An increase in neutrophils is commonly seen in CFA and inorganic dusts like asbestos. In sarcoidosis and drug-related DPLDs, an increase in lymphocytes is seen. In general, it is said that fibrosis associated with predominance of neutrophils in lavage is less responsive to steroids and hence a poorer prognosis. The prognosis is good when there is predominance of lymphocytes, for example in sarcoidosis.

Lung biopsy

This may be required if other investigations do not provide the diagnosis.

Treatment

The treatment depends on underlying pathology and usually corticosteroids alone or in combination when immunosuppressive agents like cyclophosphamide are used. Corticosteroids are helpful in conditions like sarcoidosis, hypersensitivity pneumonias, connective tissue disorders, vasculitides and cryptogenic fibrosing alveolitis. Steroids are of no benefit in inorganic dust diseases.

Patients should be advised to stop smoking. Other general measures like pneumococcal and influenza vaccination and provision of home oxygen in the presence of hypoxemia helps improve quality of life. Single lung transplantation may be considered in the advanced stage in carefully selected patients.

1.26 C
1.27 D

Lung abscess

Lung abscess is a necrotizing infection of the lung tissue leading to formation of a cavity containing pus. It usually occurs after aspiration of oral secretions in patients predisposed to aspiration.

Predisposing factors

1. *Inability to protect airway*: altered consciousness, seizures, neurological conditions with poor cough reflex, alcohol, sedation, general anaesthesia, opioids
2. *Poor oral hygiene* and gingivitis

3. *Septic emboli from other sites*: for example, tricuspid endocarditis, and bacteraemia secondary to gastrointestinal or genitourinary procedures or infections. This may cause multiple abscesses
4. *Superadded infection* on pulmonary infarct or a cavitating lung carcinoma
5. As a complication of *anaerobic pneumonias*

Causative organisms

Lung abscess is said to be caused by anaerobic organisms but in about 50% of cases both aerobic and anaerobic organisms are found. Commonly isolated pathogens are:

- *Anaerobic: Fusobacterium, Peptostreptococcus, Bacteroides* spp.
- *Aerobic: Staphylococcus aureus* (multiple abscesses may be seen), *Streptococcus pyogenes, Klebsiella, Pseudomonas, H. influenzae.*
- *Others: Mycobacterium tuberculosis, Aspergillus, Histoplasmosis.*

Clinical features

The symptoms may evolve over days to weeks. The common symptoms are lethargy, fever, weight loss, night sweats, cough, foul smelling sputum and haemoptysis. On physical examination there may be reduced air entry in the affected area, coarse inspiratory crepitations, bronchial breath sounds and dullness on percussion. Clubbing may be present.

Diagnosis

Blood tests should be arranged including full blood count, urea and electrolytes, CRP, liver function tests and glucose. The sputum should be examined for Gram stain, cytology, culture and sensitivity.

Radiology

A CXR should be obtained initially, which may show a cavity with air–fluid level. The margin of the cavity is irregular. When it appears nodular, there should be suspicion for carcinoma. If lung abscess is secondary to aspiration, the cavity is usually seen in the posterior segment of the upper lobe or superior segment of the lower lobe. In some cases there may be co-existing empyema. Multiple cavities on CXR may be due to staphylococcal or metastatic lung abscesses.

A CT scan of the chest should be obtained for further evaluation and it is helpful to rule out empyema. The abscess cavity is seen lying within the lung parenchyma and the margins may be irregular. It makes an acute angle with the chest wall.

Differential diagnosis

- Cavitating lung carcinoma
- Pulmonary cyst
- Infected bulla
- Aspergilloma
- Wegener's granulomatosis
- Hydatid cyst
- Localized empyema
- Post primary tuberculosis

Treatment

These patients need a prolonged course of antibiotics, usually for 4–6 weeks with a broad-spectrum antibiotic. The condition responds well to treatment. Advice from microbiologists should be sought regarding the choice of antibiotics. There is a risk of relapse with a shorter course of antibiotic treatment.

Some causes of treatment failure

- Underlying malignancy
- Antibiotic resistance
- Obstruction of the bronchus with foreign body
- Tuberculosis
- Debility

1.28 C
1.29 B
1.30 A

Pulmonary metastases

Malignancy can spread to the lung from a primary site mainly through the haematogenous, lymphatic route or it can be a direct extension. The primary may be from the gastrointestinal tract, kidneys, breast, melanoma, testes, thyroid, osteosarcomas, choriocarcinoma or head and neck cancers. Their detection is very important in planning the management of the primary cancer.

Clinical features

The symptoms are those of underlying primary tumour. There may not be any respiratory symptoms even in the presence of multiple metastases. Patients may develop breathlessness due to pleural effusion or obstruction of bronchus. In dyspnoea of sudden onset, pneumothorax should be ruled out.

Radiology

CXR: Pulmonary metastases are usually seen on CXR in the presence of a primary tumour. It may also be discovered incidentally. There may be solitary or multiple nodules. Solitary metastases can be seen in melanoma, colonic carcinomas and osteosarcomas. Smaller metastases can be missed on CXR. Hence, a CT scan should be carried out for further evaluation.

CT scan

The metastases are usually round in shape but may also be irregular. The size may be variable but with well-defined outline and multiple in number. They tend to occur in mostly in peripheral lung fields or at the lung bases.

The metastases from adenocarcinoma may have a lobulated appearance with an irregular outline. Metastatic squamous cell carcinoma may cavitate and have a predisposition towards upper lobes. Calcification is very uncommon and when present, other diagnoses should also be sought.

Solitary metastases are uncommon. Differentiation between primary lung cancer and metastases is important for management. Even on CT it may not be possible to differentiate between them.

Important points

- Metastases that grow very fast and bleed can have indistinct or blurry borders, e.g. choriocarcinoma.
- Calcification in lung metastases is unusual, except for chondrosarcoma, osteosarcoma.
- *Abscopal effect*: spontaneous resolution of lung secondaries when primary is treated, e.g. renal cell carcinoma and trophoblastic tumours.
- Trophoblastic tumours and thyroid cancer can give rise to a snowstorm appearance on CXR.

Lymphangitis carcinomatosis

This is the invasion of the pulmonary lymphatics with the tumour cells and can be seen in bronchial, breast, pancreatic, stomach or prostate cancer. The usual symptoms are dry cough and breathlessness, and carry a bad prognosis.

The CXR may show reticulo-nodular shadowing with or without thickening of the interlobular septae. There may also be thickening of the lung fissures. The findings are usually bilateral but can be unilateral as in bronchial carcinoma. A pleural effusion may be present. It may mimic pulmonary oedema or lung fibrosis.

Sometimes the CXR may appear normal. HRCT is the imaging modality of choice if the condition is suspected and also for further evaluation.

Differential diagnosis

Solitary nodule

- Lung carcinoma
- Tuberculosis
- Wegener's granulomatosis
- Lung abscess
- Hamartoma
- Round pneumonia

Multiple nodules

- Metastatic cancer
- Metastatic abscesses
- Histoplasmosis
- Wegener's granulomatosis
- Sarcoidosis

1.31 B
1.32 D

Round pneumonia

Round pneumonia is a clinical entity that can be easily confused with bronchogenic carcinoma. It appears as a coin lesion on CXR and it is often misinterpreted as a malignancy. It mainly involves small bronchi and alveoli. There is usually multisegment involvement but spread to adjacent lobes is confined by interlobar septae. The organisms commonly involved are *Klebsiella, Streptococcus pneumoniae* and *Mycobacterium tuberculosis*.

Clinical features
Round pneumonia is more commonly seen in children but is also seen in adults. The symptoms can be mild. The usual symptoms are fever, chills and cough. A history of febrile illness goes more in favour of an infective process than malignancy although this may not be always true. There is symptomatic improvement with antibiotics and with resolution of the opacity on the CXR.

Diagnosis
The WCC is raised and CRP or ESR may be elevated. If there is sputum production it should be sent for culture.

Radiology
A CXR should be obtained initially. A round or oval opacity is seen. The margins can be smooth or they may be irregular. The opacity is mainly seen in the lower lobe and if it is in the upper lobe, it is more likely to be malignant. Air bronchograms can be present but are not characteristic, as they can also be seen in malignancy.

CT scan is helpful for further evaluation. A heterogeneous mass of soft tissue attenuation is seen. It may appear spiculated and air bronchograms may be present. Satellite lesions, if present, are an important finding. In peripherally located lesions pleural thickening may be present.

Treatment
The patients should be treated with a course of antibiotics and the repeat CXR should be obtained to look for resolution.

1.33 C
1.34 A
1.35 C

Pneumocystis carinii pneumonia

Pneumocystis carinii (now called *Pneumocystis jiroveci*) is an opportunistic fungal pathogen. *Pneumocystis carinii* pneumonia (PCP) is the most common opportunistic infection occurring in patients with HIV infection and in other immunocompromised patients. It carries higher mortality rate in non-HIV than in patients with HIV infection. The mortality also tends to rise when there is a delay in starting treatment.

Predisposing factors
- HIV patients with CD4 count of < 200/μL and not on PCP prophylaxis
- Patients receiving immunosuppressive agents, for example transplant recipients and those with collagen vascular disorders
- Those with congenital immunodeficiency states, for example hypogammaglobulinaemia
- Those with haematological malignancies

Clinical features

The usual symptoms are dry cough, breathlessness on exertion, weight loss, malaise and fever. The patients may have tachypnoea, tachycardia, and cyanosis and on chest auscultation fine crepitations may be heard or it may sound normal. There may be other associated extrapulmonary features like hepatomegaly and lymphadenopathy, although they are rare.

Diagnosis

Blood tests: there may be leucocytosis and lymphopaenia. LDH is usually elevated. It has high sensitivity but low specificity. The levels should improve with treatment and if they don't, it implies a bad prognosis. There is hypoxemia and respiratory alkalosis on ABG analysis. The degree of hypoxemia can be an indicator of prognosis. There is an increase in alveolar to arterial oxygen gradient (PA_{O2}–Pa_{O2}). The severity can be graded according to the level of hypoxemia and the PA_{O2}–Pa_{O2} gradient into mild, moderate and severe types.

Sputum: diagnosis can be made by demonstration of *Pneumocystis* in the sputum sample obtained by inhalation of hypertonic saline. This is a non-invasive method and has high specificity.

Bronchoalveolar lavage (BAL): this should be done if sputum induction is not possible and is usually diagnostic. It may be less useful in patients with a relapse. Transbronchial biopsy is rarely needed to establish a diagnosis.

Pulmonary function tests (PFTs): the diffusion capacity for carbon monoxide (TLCO) is reduced. In patients with normal TLCO and normal HRCT, PCP is unlikely.

Radiology

CXR findings include bilateral, diffuse, reticular infiltrates that begin in the perihilar region and may progress to diffuse airspace consolidation. Less commonly patchy infiltrates may be seen. In patients using aerosolized pentamidine the infiltrates may be seen in the upper lobes. In some cases the CXR may appear normal. The CXR may also show pneumatoceles. Spontaneous pneumothorax, which can be bilateral, is a recognized complication of PCP and the risk increases in the presence of pneumatoceles. Pneumothorax can also occur in association with use of inhaled pentamidine. The pneumothoraces in association with PCP may be very difficult to treat.

HRCT is very sensitive and is helpful when a CXR is normal. The usual finding is of bilateral ground-glass attenuation, which may give it a mosaic appearance. There may be interlobular septal thickening. A negative HRCT does not rule out PCP.

Gallium 67 scan shows increased uptake in PCP but has limited role. It may be useful in suspected relapse as BAL may be less useful in these cases.

Differential diagnosis

- *Mycoplasma* infection

- Acute respiratory distress syndrome (ARDS)
- Pulmonary oedema
- Tuberculosis
- Cryptogenic organizing pneumonia
- Hypersensitivity pneumonitis
- Metastatic disease

Treatment
Intravenous co-trimoxazole (trimethoprim and sulphamethoxazole) is the drug of choice. The duration of treatment is for 21 days in HIV and 14 days in non-HIV patients. Patients should be advised to stop smoking. Prophylaxis with co-trimoxazole should be given to those with CD4 count of < 200/μL, a history of oral thrush and to all the patients with prior history of PCP. Aerosolized pentamidine is an alternative but is less effective and there is a risk of patients developing pneumothorax.

1.36 C
1.37 B
1.38 C

Drug-induced lung disease

Drug-induced lung disease poses a diagnostic challenge as clinical and radiological findings are non-specific. A careful history is of paramount importance. The drug reactions can be immune-mediated, when the outcome is usually good, or it can be due to cytotoxic effect leading to fibrosis, when the prognosis is poor.

The patterns of drug-induced lung disease may fall into four broad types:

- Interstitial pneumonitis and fibrosis
- Hypersensitivity reaction
- ARDS
- Cryptogenic organizing pneumonia

Two more types may be seen: pulmonary haemorrhage (seen with anticoagulants and salicylates) and eosinophilic pneumonia.

Clinical features
These are non-specific. In acute hypersensitivity reactions the patients may present with fever, dry cough, dyspnoea and this may be associated with a rash. The onset may be insidious in patients with pulmonary fibrosis and they usually present with breathlessness on exertion. Chest auscultatory findings can be variable depending on the underlying pathology.

Diagnosis
It can be difficult as the findings are non-specific and hence the importance of good history. Usually a combination of clinical, radiological and histopathology findings are needed to arrive at a diagnosis.

Blood tests may show elevated WCC and there may be associated eosinophilia. The lung function tests may show a restrictive pattern. The imaging procedures may not be diagnostic of one particular offending agent but the pattern and the distribution of the disease can help narrow the differentials. The patients may require BAL or a lung biopsy.

Radiology

A CXR should be obtained initially. HRCT is superior to CXR and should be done if CXR is normal or equivocal. The radiographic findings include:

- Linear or reticulonodular opacities may be seen or a bilateral mixed airspace and interstitial pattern.
- There may be patchy areas of consolidation.
- In pulmonary fibrosis bilateral, reticular and linear shadowing in the lung bases are seen.

Based on the type of drug reaction, the HRCT findings may be one of the following:

1. Interstitial pneumonitis and fibrosis:
   - Ground-glass opacities, focal areas of consolidation and irregular linear opacities mainly in the lower zone of the lungs.
   - Examples include chemotherapeutic agents like bleomycin, methotrexate and nitrofurantoin.
2. Hypersensitivity reaction:
   - Ground-glass opacities and poorly defined centrilobular nodules. Also extensive bilateral airspace consolidation may be seen.
   - Example: methotrexate.
3. ARDS:
   - Bilateral dependent air-space consolidation
   - The onset is usually sudden.
   - Examples: heroin, cocaine, salicylate toxicity, phenylbutazone
4. Cryptogenic organizing pneumonia:
   - Peribronchial or subpleural areas of consolidation
   - Examples: bleomycin, amiodarone, nitrofurantoin

Differential diagnosis

- Tuberculosis
- Sarcoidosis
- *Pneumocystis carinii* pneumonia
- Interstitial pneumonia
- Metastatic carcinoma

Treatment

This depends on the underlying pathology. The mainstay of the treatment is withdrawal of the offending agent and in some cases steroids are beneficial.

Important points

- Pleural effusion is uncommon in drug-induced lung disease but can be seen with drugs causing systemic lupus-like syndrome. Examples: procainamide, sulphonamides, methyldopa, hydralazine and isoniazid. There is no renal involvement in lupus-like syndrome caused by drugs.

- Hilar or mediastinal lymphadenopathy is not seen except with anti-convulsants like phenytoin and methotrexate.
- Nodules in the lung may develop with bleomycin therapy that may be confused with metastases.
- Treatment with nitrosoureas may cause pneumothorax.
- Drugs causing eosinophilia with pulmonary infiltrates – nitrofurantoin, tetracycline, penicillin, sulfasalazine.

1.39 B
1.40 A
1.41 B

Pneumothorax

Pneumothorax is accumulation of air in the pleural space. It is more common in males than females and is usually seen in young, tall and thin males. When it occurs in healthy lungs it is called primary pneumothorax (PSP) and when it occurs in pre-existing lung disease it is called secondary pneumothorax (SSP). Subpleural blebs are thought to be the underlying aetiological factor in primary pneumothorax.

Classification

1. Spontaneous: primary or secondary
2. Traumatic
3. Iatrogenic

Some causes of secondary pneumothorax:

- COPD/asthma
- Pulmonary infections like TB, pneumonias
- Diffuse pulmonary lung disease
- Hereditary conditions like Marfan's syndrome

Catamenial pneumothorax
This term is used when pneumothorax occurs in menstruating women. It is usually but not invariably associated with endometriosis. It occurs commonly in women in their fourth decade. It can be recurrent and is more common on the right side.

Clinical features
Patients may present with chest pain or dyspnoea. The chest pain may be sharp and/or pleuritic in nature. In PSP, the symptoms may resolve after 1–2 days even though the pneumothorax persists. In SSP, the patients may be severely dyspnoeic due to underlying lung disease and the symptoms do not improve.

On physical examination, there is reduced air entry or absent breath sounds on the affected side. The chest movement is diminished and the percussion note is hyper-resonant. In SSP, the clinical signs may not be prominent due to underlying lung disease.

Diagnosis

Arterial blood gases may show reduced PCO_2 and respiratory alkalosis. Hypoxemia is seen particularly in patients with underlying lung disease.

Radiology

A CXR should be obtained initially but is less sensitive than a CT scan. The pneumothorax is visible when the air in the pleural space rises to the apex. The margin of visceral pleura is seen separate from the chest wall with an area of hyperlucency and loss of vascular markings. Sometimes artefacts like skin folds or clothing may appear as lung margin. If in doubt, the CXR should be repeated or a CXR with breath held in expiration may be helpful. A CT scan is particularly helpful for further evaluation.

The CT is helpful to differentiate between bullae or a pneumothorax. Also, apical subpleural blebs may be seen. It may give information about underlying lung pathology and can identify loculated pneumothorax. A CT is also helpful when CXR does not provide much information in the presence of surgical emphysema or when aberrant tube placement is suspected.

The pneumothoraces can be divided into small (< 2 cm) or large (> 2 cm).

Treatment

- Patients with a small pneumothorax and minimal symptoms can be observed.
- Aspiration should be tried first in PSP requiring intervention.
- Aspiration should only be tried in SSP when the size is small with minimal breathlessness. These patients should be observed for at least 24 hours afterwards.
- Intercostal tube drainage should be done when aspiration has proved unsuccessful, the patient is symptomatic or having SSP.

Complications of pneumothorax

- Tension pneumothorax
- Re-expansion pulmonary oedema
- Pyopneumothorax
- Recurrence either on same or contralateral side
- Pneumomediastinum

Important points

- Pneumothorax is a recognized complication of nebulized pentamidine therapy.
- In PCP, pneumothorax carries a high mortality rate and it may not resolve with intercostal tube drainage.
- It is a complication of metastatic sarcomas.
- It also occurs frequently with histiocytosis X and lymphangioleiomyomatosis.

Section 2: Abdomen

Questions

2.1 A 56-year-old man who is known to have cirrhosis of the liver secondary to excessive alcohol consumption presents with increased abdominal pain and ascites. A CT scan of his abdomen is shown. You suspect hepatocellular carcinoma. What investigation is most helpful?

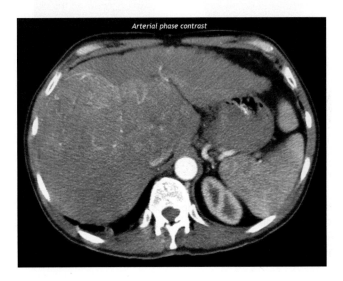

Arterial phase contrast

A. Diagnostic aspiration of the ascitic fluid, looking for cancer cells
B. AFP levels
C. MRI of the liver
D. Liver biopsy

2.2 All the following are true regarding hepatocellular carcinoma (HCC) except:

A. AFP is always elevated.
B. Acquired porphyria may be a feature of HCC.
C. Ultrasound has same sensitivity as CT in detecting HCC.
D. Liver transplantation may be an option for solitary tumours < 5 cm.

2.3 A 58-year-old man presented with painful dysphagia, poor appetite and weight loss. He is a heavy smoker and also drinks alcohol excessively. An urgent barium swallow was arranged and is shown. What is the most likely diagnosis?

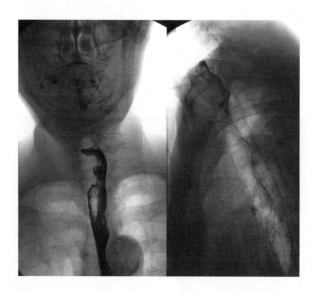

A. Adenocarcinoma of the oesophagus
B. Achalasia cardia
C. Oesophageal dysmotility
D. Squamous cell carcinoma of the oesophagus

2.4 All of the following are true regarding carcinoma of the oesophagus except:

A. Hypercalcaemia may be seen in squamous cell carcinoma.
B. On staging CT if a tumour is seen encircling aorta it is more likely to be a squamous cell carcinoma.
C. In chronic reflux, carcinoma of the oesophagus arises only in presence of Barrett's oesophagus.
D. EUS is superior to CT in assessing local invasion.

2.5 A 30-year-old woman presented with a history of abdominal pain, weight loss and diarrhoea and also complained of having recurrent mouth ulcers and redness of her eyes. She is a smoker and her past medical history includes treatment for anal fissure and ischiorectal abscess. A small bowel barium study was carried out and is shown. What is the most likely diagnosis?

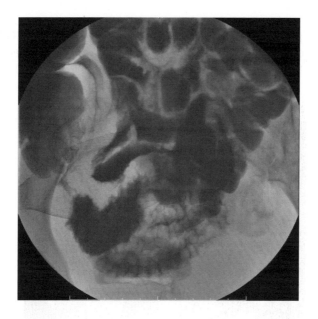

A. Tuberculosis
B. Carcinoid syndrome
C. Crohn's disease
D. Lymphoma

2.6   All the following are radiological features of Crohn's disease on small bowel meal except:

A. Granular mucosa
B. Aphthoid ulcers
C. String sign of Kantor
D. Cobblestone appearance

2.7   In relation to Crohn's disease, all the following are true except:

A. String sign of Kantor on small bowel enema is usually caused by spasm in the small intestine.
B. Toxic dilatation of the colon is extremely common.
C. Multiple strictures on small bowel meal are very suggestive of Crohn's disease.
D. The most common finding on CT is thickening of the bowel wall.

2.8 A 60-year-old woman presented with symptoms of poor appetite, weight loss, sweating and abdominal discomfort. An ultrasound of the abdomen and CT scan are shown and metastatic disease to liver is suspected. Of the following the most uncommon primary site would be:

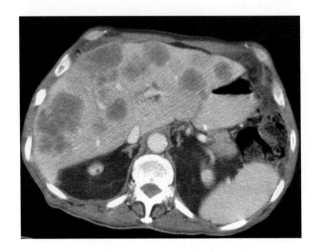

A. Melanoma
B. Lung
C. Breast
D. Stomach

2.9 All the following are true except:

A. MRI is more sensitive than CT in detecting hepatic metastases.
B. Mucinous adenocarcinomas may give rise to calcified metastases.
C. The pattern of metastatic lesions on ultrasound usually does not specify the primary site of origin of the tumour.
D. The tumour cells from the GI tract reach the liver mostly through the portal vein.

2.10 A 60-year-old woman presented with complaints of retrosternal chest pain and dysphagia. An urgent barium swallow was arranged and is shown. For the condition shown, what investigation would you arrange to confirm the diagnosis?

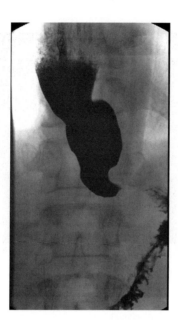

A. Upper GI endoscopy
B. CT scan
C. Oesophageal manometry
D. Combination of manometry and upper GI endoscopy

2.11 All the following are true of achalasia except:

A. Absence of stomach gas bubble on chest X-ray
B. 'Bird beak' appearance on the barium swallow
C. Barium swallow helps to rule out achalasia even in very early stages
D. Oesophageal fluid level may be seen on chest X-ray

2.12 A 55-year-old man who is a known alcoholic has pancreatitis. He started having swinging pyrexia, vomiting and hiccups. His liver was palpable and there was dullness on percussion over the right lower thoracic cage. A CT scan was arranged and is shown. What is the most likely diagnosis given the clinical scenario and CT findings?

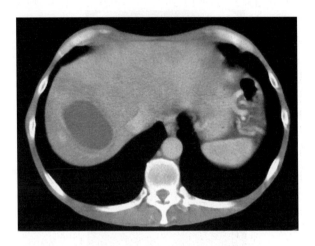

A. Metastatic carcinoma
B. Liver abscess
C. Empyema
D. Perforated abdominal viscus

2.13 All of the following are true of liver abscess except:

A. Amoebic serology is positive in 90–95% of patients.
B. A prolonged course of high-dose intravenous antibiotics usually cures the condition.
C. ALP is elevated most of the time.
D. Contrast CT is preferable to MRI to help with diagnosis and further evaluation.

2.14 This 32-year-old woman had presented with symptoms of right upper quadrant discomfort and abdominal distension. She was a known smoker and is known to be having inflammatory bowel disease which was poorly controlled. On clinical examination she appeared slightly jaundiced and was found to be having ascites. A CT scan of the abdomen was done (shown) and you suspect Budd-Chiari syndrome. Please choose the correct response:

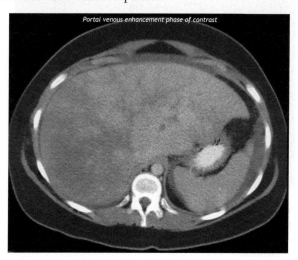

Portal venous enhancement phase of contrast

A. MRI is the most useful investigation to confirm the diagnosis.
B. Hepatic venography is used as gold standard.
C. CT confirms the diagnosis and no other investigation may be required.
D. The CT scan almost always can detect thrombus in the hepatic vein.

2.15 All the following are true regarding Budd-Chiari syndrome except:

A. The acute type is most commonly seen.
B. Serum-ascites albumin gradient of > 1.1.
C. Caudate lobe enlargement on CT is suggestive of Budd-Chiari syndrome.
D. Hepatic venous webs are best demonstrated on hepatic venography.

2.16 A 55-year-old man presented with a history of abdominal pain, weight loss and fever. His BP was recorded to be high at 170/110 mmHg. He is a known smoker and is on dialysis for end-stage renal disease (ESRD). A CT scan of his abdomen is shown. What is the most likely diagnosis?

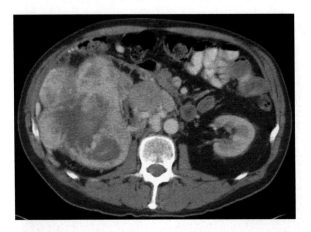

A. Renal cell carcinoma
B. Lymphoma
C. Transitional cell carcinoma
D. Wilm's tumour

2.17 All the following are true of renal cell carcinoma except:

A. The varicocele is usually seen on the left side.
B. CT scan is the imaging modality of choice for detection and staging of the tumour.
C. The classical triad of loin pain, haematuria and abdominal or flank mass is seen in only 80–90% of patients on presentation.
D. Hepatic dysfunction (Stauffer's syndrome) seen in renal cell carcinoma improves with treatment.

2.18 A 55-year-old woman presented with complaints of malaise, pain in the right hypochondrium and poor appetite. She was also jaundiced. Her liver function tests showed raised ALP and ALT. A CT scan of the abdomen was carried out and is shown. What is the most likely diagnosis?

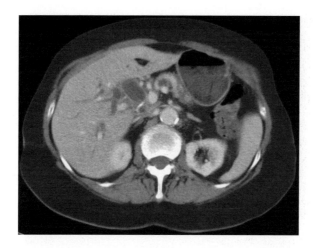

A. Obstructive jaundice
B. Acute pancreatitis
C. Acute hepatitis
D. Acute cholecystitis

2.19 All the following are true except:

A. When the gallbladder is palpable it implies CBD obstruction may be secondary to carcinoma of the head of the pancreas.
B. The sensitivity of Ultrasound is 100% in presence of CBD stones.
C. When obstruction is removed from the CBD, ALT is first to improve.
D. A CT scan always identifies the CBD stones.

2.20 A 35-year-old man, who is a known alcoholic, presented with severe abdominal pain, vomiting and fever. His blood pressure was 86/48 and his serum amylase levels were > 1000 u/mL. A CT scan was carried out and is shown. Acute pancreatitis is suspected. Please choose the correct statement:

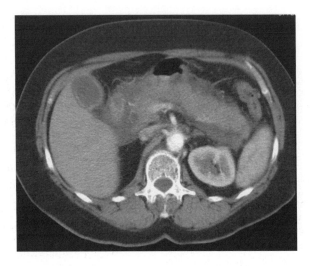

A. A pleural effusion, if present, is usually right sided.
B. The abdominal pain improves on lying supine.
C. Turner's sign, when present, implies a poor prognosis.
D. Pancreatic pseudocyst develops typically 8–10 weeks after onset of symptoms.

2.21 All the following are true except:

A. Pancreatitis may be missed on ultrasound in about 15–20% cases.
B. CT scan of the abdomen should be done immediately on presentation.
C. MRCP helps to detect CBD or pancreatic duct stricture.
D. The CT scan can be delayed to 48–72 hours after onset of symptoms.

Section 2: Abdomen

Answers

2.1 B
2.2 A

Hepatocellular carcinoma

Heptatocellular carcinoma (HCC) is a very common cancer and is the most common primary liver cancer. It is more common in Asia and Africa but less common in the western world. It is more common in males than females.

Risk factors
Cirrhosis of the liver is a major risk factor and is more common in the macronodular type. It can be associated with any condition leading to chronic liver disease and cirrhosis. Some of the causes are mentioned below:

- Hepatitis B or C infection
- Alcoholic liver disease
- Haemochromatosis
- Primary biliary cirrhosis
- α-1 anti-trypsin deficiency
- Non-alcoholic steatohepatitis (NASH)
- Aflatoxin

Clinical features

- Abdominal pain
- Ascites
- Jaundice

HCC should be suspected if the above symptoms develop in a patient known to have cirrhosis of the liver. HCC may spread to adjacent structures and may metastasize to lungs or bones.
Other features of HCC are:

- Polycythaemia
- Hypoglycaemia
- Hypercalcaemia
- Hypercholesterolaemia
- Polymyositis
- Acquired porphyria

Diagnosis
ALP and AFP levels are elevated. AFP is elevated in 80% of patients but HCC can also occur with normal AFP. Ultrasound of the liver can detect the tumour and it has same sensitivity as CT. Presence of tumour on ultrasound and an AFP level of > 400 ng/mL is highly suggestive of HCC. Liver biopsy may be needed when multiple lesions are seen but it should be avoided when

the tumour is confined to one lobe of the liver. The ascitic fluid cytology to detect cancer cells is not usually helpful.

Radiology

HCC can be of solitary, multicentric or diffuse type. Once the tumour is seen on ultrasound, further evaluation with a CT or MRI is required.

The unenhanced CT scan shows an area of reduced attenuation. HCC is a hypervascular tumour and contrast CT shows enhancement in the arterial phase. It enhances heterogeneously (mosaic pattern), the margins may be irregular and a capsule may be seen. The smaller lesions may appear homogeneous. The lesions appear heterogeneous on MRI. On T1-weighted images there is reduced signal intensity and on T2-weighted images increased signal is seen.

Differential diagnosis

- Focal nodular hyperplasia
- Metastases
- Haemangioma

Treatment

Surgical resection offers definitive cure but usually the tumour is quite advanced on presentation and resection is not possible. The tumour should be confined to one lobe. There is a risk of recurrence. Liver transplantation may be an option for those with a single tumour of < 5 cm or three tumours < 3 cm in size. Chemotherapy alone is not very effective. The other available options are hepatic artery embolization and chemotherapy, radiofrequency ablation, and ultrasound-guided ethanol injection. In all patients with cirrhosis monitoring should be carried out by ultrasound and AFP levels checked every 6 months.

Some other causes of a raised AFP are:

- Hepatitis
- Metastases from stomach and colon
- Pregnancy
- Testicular or pancreatic tumours

2.3 B
2.4 A

Carcinoma of the oesophagus

Oesophageal carcinoma is a relatively uncommon but highly malignant cancer and carries a very poor prognosis because by the time the patients are symptomatic the disease is quite advanced. It is commoner in males than females and the prevalence is higher in lower socioeconomic groups. It is of two types: squamous cell carcinoma and adenocarcinoma.

Risk factors

- *Squamous cell carcinoma*: smoking, excessive alcohol consumption (risk higher with spirits), achalasia, strictures secondary to radiation, Plummer-Vinson syndrome and nitrate ingestion.

- *Adenocarcinoma*: Owing to chronic acid reflux, the squamous epithelium changes to columnar-lined oesophagus (CLO, also called Barrett's oesophagus). This may undergo various degrees of dysplasia to change into adenocarcinoma, but oesophageal cancer can also arise in chronic reflux without progressing to CLO.

Plummer-Vinson syndrome

This syndrome consists of anaemia, glossitis and oesophageal web.

Clinical features

About 50% of the oesophageal cancers develop in the lower third. The commonest symptom is dysphagia, which is initially to solids and later also to liquids. This may be associated with pain (odynophagia). There may be weight loss, poor appetite, nausea or vomiting. The patients may also develop aspiration pneumonia. New-onset dysphagia on the background of longstanding reflux symptoms merits urgent investigations. It may metastasize to liver, lungs and regional lymph nodes.

Diagnosis

When the condition is suspected, an urgent barium swallow is a useful initial investigation. Upper GI endoscopy should be done urgently and biopsies taken along with brushings from the tumour. A staging CT scan of the thorax, abdomen and pelvis along with endoluminal ultrasound should be arranged. Baseline blood tests including calcium levels should be carried out. Hypercalcaemia may be present in squamous cell carcinoma. If surgery is planned, an ECG, echocardiography and lung function tests are also required.

Radiology

The initial barium swallow gives useful information on the morphology of the tumour and the motility of the oesophagus. The mucosa appears irregular and narrowing or constriction may be seen. The lesion may appear as a polypoid mass or ulcerating growth.

The staging CT provides valuable information on local invasion, lymph node involvement and metastases to liver or lung. Thickening of the oesophageal wall is seen, which is irregular, and the oesophagus may be dilated, with presence of fluid and debris above the lesion. Furthermore, the relationship of the tumour to the neighbouring structures like the aorta may be defined, as squamous cell carcinoma has a tendency to grow towards the aorta; it may be seen encircling the aorta.

The endoscopic ultrasound (EUS) helps to visualize local invasion as it can demonstrate all the layers of the wall of the oesophagus and should be routinely performed along with CT or MRI. EUS is better than CT or MRI in assessing mural invasion. The positron-emission tomography (PET) scan is also increasingly used by oncologists in detecting and following up the tumour.

Differential diagnosis

- Achalasia cardia
- Benign oesophageal stricture
- Schatki ring
- Leiomyoma
- Oesophageal varices

Treatment

When surgical resection is not possible due to advanced disease, which is usually the case as the disease is advanced on presentation, palliative care should be the aim. Relief of dysphagia in the form of endoscopic dilatation may be required. In only 45% of patients is surgery possible but residual tumour may be there in the margins of the resected specimen. Chemotherapy may help reduce the tumour size. A combination of chemotherapy and radiotherapy on their own or as a neoadjuvant treatment prior to the surgery is also used.

2.5 C
2.6 A
2.7 B

Crohn's disease

Crohn's disease (CD) is a condition of unknown aetiology and is characterized by transmural inflammation and presence of granulomas microscopically. It may involve any area of the GI tract from the mouth to the anus but the terminal ileum is most commonly involved. The rectum is spared typically. The inflammation is segmental (skip lesions) and the patients tend to develop fistulae, fissures and strictures. The condition is more common in smokers and smoking increases the risk of relapse.

Clinical features

The symptoms of CD depend on the type and location of the disease. The common symptoms are diarrhoea and abdominal pain. There may be a history of weight loss. A low-grade pyrexia, anorexia, nausea, vomiting and nutritional deficiencies may also be seen. Patients may present with perianal fistulating disease and anal stenosis. A high temperature may indicate intra-abdominal abscess formation. There are some extraintestinal manifestations that are indicative of active inflammation and these include mouth ulcers, episcleritis and iritis, arthritis, sacroiliitis and erythema nodosum. The granulomas may also be seen in the liver and pancreas and there may be associated fatty infiltration of the liver.

Diagnosis

The aim of the investigations should be to establish the diagnosis, to define the type and extent of the disease and to detect associated complications.

The blood tests may show anaemia, leucocytosis, raised CRP or ESR, and low albumin; abnormal liver function signs may be seen. There may be vitamin and mineral deficiencies, e.g. vitamin B_{12}, folic acid, vitamin D, iron, calcium, magnesium and trace elements.

Small bowel meal and follow-through is a useful initial investigation in patients with symptoms suggestive of small bowel disease. A CT or MRI may be required for evaluation of abscesses or fistulating disease. In the presence of diarrhoea or rectal bleeding, colonoscopy is preferable to barium enema. This will also allow for biopsies to be taken, which will help with diagnosis. A plain X-ray of the abdomen should also be obtained. Toxic dilatation of the colon (> 6 cm) is more common in ulcerative colitis than CD.

Radiology

The barium examination of the small bowel may show aphthoid ulcers, fissure ulcers or longitudinal ulcers. The fissure ulcers may cause fistulae or abscess formation. A cobblestone appearance due to longitudinal and transverse ulcers with normal mucosa in between may also be seen, particularly in the terminal ileum. Narrowing of the lumen of the small bowel and strictures may be seen. In fact, multiple strictures are strongly indicative of CD. Sometimes narrowing of the small bowel lumen due to spasm is seen (string sign of Kantor) and this may not be due to stenosis of the small bowel.

On CT scan thickening of the small bowel wall is seen most commonly. The CT may also demonstrate serosal abnormalities, abscesses, mesenteric inflammation and lymphadenopathy.

Ultrasound may be a useful investigation to look for small intestinal wall abnormalities, masses and abscesses. It can also be used to assess the response to treatment. ^{99}Tcm-HMPAO leucocyte scan can help exclude active CD and may help localize abscesses.

Differential diagnosis of small bowel stricture

- Tuberculosis
- Carcinoma
- Actinomycosis
- Lymphoma
- Carcinoid syndrome
- Strongyloidosis

Treatment

- A multidisciplinary team approach is required. Close co-operation between gastroenterologists, surgeons and dietitians is required. Good nutritional support is paramount in addition to the available treatment modalities. Full information on the condition should be provided to the patient.
- *Medical management*: this usually consists of use of aminosalicylates (e.g. mesalazine, balsalazide) for maintenance of remission and courses of oral steroids (prednisolone) may be needed if there are flare-ups. Immunomodulating agents like azathioprine may be required as steroid sparing agents. For severe flare-ups, admission to hospital with intravenous hydrocortisone, metronidazole may be required. Infliximab is used in severe CD or in fistulating disease.
- *Surgical treatment*: about 70–75% patients with CD may require surgery at some point. It is usually needed in steroid-resistant CD, treatment of local complications or intestinal obstruction.

Complications of CD

- Abscesses/fistulae/anal fissure
- Intestinal obstruction
- Perforation
- Short-gut syndrome
- Bacterial overgrowth and bile salt malabsorption

- Primary sclerosing cholangitis
- Carcinoma
- Osteoporosis/osteomalacia
- Hyperoxaluria and nephrolithiasis

Associations of CD

- Turner's syndrome
- Selective IgA deficiency
- Hereditary angioedema
- Hermansky–Pudlak syndrome

2.8 D
2.9 A

Hepatic metastases

The liver is one of the organs most commonly affected by metastatic disease and it is the second most commonly involved organ after the lymph nodes. Cancer from any primary site can metastasize to the liver with the exception of the primary brain neoplasm. The metastases are usually haematogenous in origin. The cancers from the GI tract reach the liver via the portal vein and from other primary sites through the hepatic artery. Most commonly metastases are from the GI tract (colon, stomach, and pancreas), lung, breast and malignant melanoma, and the uncommon sites of a primary tumour are prostate, thyroid etc. In most cases there are multiple metastatic lesions. Occasionally only a solitary lesion may be seen and on rare circumstances a diffuse pattern is seen.

Some other characteristics of the metastases include:

- When the malignancy has spread to the liver it may also have spread to the other sites like lungs or bones except for colonic carcinoma and carcinoid, when they may be confined to the liver.
- Most metastases may be hypovascular with exceptions being neuroendocrine tumours, renal cell carcinoma, choriocarcinoma, thyroid carcinoma or carcinoids.
- With some metastases calcification may be seen that may appear amorphous or granular.

Clinical features
They may be of the underlying primary tumour and symptoms related to the hepatic metastases may be non-specific. The patients may have low-grade pyrexia, sweating, weight loss, and poor appetite. There may be right upper quadrant discomfort or pain. Ascites may be present, which may indicate a poor prognosis. The liver may be palpable and it may appear nodular. There may be obstruction to the bile ducts leading to obstructive jaundice.

Diagnosis
The liver function tests may be abnormal but are non-specific. Elevation of ALP is more commonly seen and ALT may also be mildly elevated. Other blood abnormalities include anaemia, leucocytosis and low albumin.

Amongst the biochemical markers for liver function, elevation in 5-nucleoti-dase is the most sensitive.

Radiology
Ultrasound is a very good initial investigation and is very sensitive though the pattern of metastases is quite varied and may not be able to specify the primary site. The lesions may appear hypoechoic or hyperechoic. A target or bull's eye pattern may be seen. Large or moderately sized hyperechoic lesions may be seen with colonic cancer.

Contrast-enhanced CT is very sensitive in detecting hepatic metastases (80–90%). The metastatic lesions appear as areas of reduced attenuation. Rim enhancement may be seen. Calcification may be detected and an area of central necrosis may be seen within the tumour.

MRI has equal sensitivity to that of CT and is usually used as a problem-solving modality. On MRI the metastases appear as areas of reduced attenuation on T1-weighted images and increased signal on T2-weighted images. Contrast-enhanced images may show similar appearance to that of CT; the exception is metastatic melanoma, which may appear as increased intensity in T1-weighted images. The haemangioma may be confused with metastases and MRI can resolve this issue.

Treatment
Once hepatic metastases are detected the prognosis is very poor. The median survival is usually only 2–4 months. The aim should be palliation to help reduce the symptoms and to improve the quality of life. Systemic chemotherapy may help reduce the tumour bulk and its growth but do not improve the prognosis. Occasionally, surgical resection may be possible for a solitary metastasis. Other measures include intrahepatic chemotherapy, radiofrequency ablation and chemoembolization.

Causes of calcified liver metastases

- Mucinous adenocarcinoma of the stomach or pancreas
- Neuroblastoma
- Medullary carcinoma of the thyroid
- Leiomyosarcoma of the stomach
- Chondrosarcoma

2.10 D
2.11 C

Achalasia cardia

Achalasia cardia is a condition of unknown aetiology. It occurs due to degeneration of the myenteric plexus. It leads to high pressure in the lower oesophageal sphincter (LOS) and is associated with its failure to relax on swallowing. There is also reduced or absent peristaltic movement.

Clinical features
The most common presenting symptom is dysphagia either to solids or to liquids. There may be pain on swallowing (odynophagia) or retrosternal dis-

comfort or chest pain on eating. The patient may also regurgitate undigested food and this increases the risk of aspiration. Other features that may be present include weight loss and poor appetite. The symptoms may be precipitated by cold liquids or stress. With longstanding achalasia there is a risk of developing squamous cell carcinoma.

Diagnosis
An upper GI endoscopy helps to visualize the oesophagus directly to identify any other lesions mimicking achalasia, and to rule out strictures and also carcinoma of the cardia. A chest X-ray and barium swallow under fluoroscopic guidance should be arranged. Oesophageal manometry helps to differentiate between achalasia and oesophageal spasm and a combination of manometry and upper GI endoscopy helps to confirm the diagnosis.

Radiology
A chest X-ray shows the absence of a stomach gas bubble and the oesophageal fluid level may be seen. It may also help identify signs of aspiration. A barium swallow may show the typical 'bird beak' appearance of the gastro-oesophageal junction. The oesophagus may appear dilated with the presence of food debris. The barium swallow may not be helpful to rule out achalasia in its earlier stages.

Differential diagnosis

- Diffuse oesophageal spasm
- Carcinoma of the cardia
- Gastric lymphoma
- Chagas' disease
- Systemic sclerosis

Treatment

- *Medical treatment:* pharmacological agents like calcium channel blockers and nitrates may help relax the LOS.
- *Botulinum toxin injection* is effective only for a few months and is not commonly used. However this may be an option for patients not able to undergo surgery.
- *Pneumatic balloon dilatation:* repeated dilatations are usually required and it carries a risk of perforation of the oesophagus.
- *Oesophageal* myotomy is effective in about 90% of patients and nowadays is being performed laparoscopically.

2.12 B
2.13 B

Liver abscess

Liver abscess is a relatively uncommon condition but can be fatal if left unrecognized and untreated. With improvement in the diagnostic techniques the mortality rates have improved.

The following types may be seen:

- *Pyogenic* (the commonest). This is due to infection in the pelvic region or peritoneum or to inflammatory bowel disease. It most commonly arises secondary to biliary tract disease (usually Gram-negative bacilli and enterococci), pancreatitis, suppurative thrombophlebitis of the portal vein due to infection in the pelvic region, inflammatory bowel disease or peritoneum
- *Haematogenous*, e.g. from infective endocarditis, pyelonephritis
- *Secondary to penetrating injuries*
- *Amoebic abscess* seen in endemic areas or in travellers to these areas
- *Abscesses caused by Candida* in immunocompromised and neutropaenic individuals
- *Cryptogenic*

Clinical features
Fever is the most common symptom and there may be abdominal signs like guarding and localized tenderness in the right hypochondrium. There may be associated symptoms like loss of appetite, rigors, cough, hiccups and vomiting. The elderly may present with pyrexia of unknown origin. Hepatomegaly and jaundice is seen in only 50% of patients. Tenderness on percussion or a friction rub may be heard on auscultation and chest signs relating to the right lower zone may be present.

Diagnosis
Blood tests may show anaemia, leucocytosis and raised CRP or ESR. Amongst liver function tests ALP is most commonly raised. Serum bilirubin may be elevated along with ALT. Serum albumin levels may be low. Blood cultures should be obtained though they are positive in only about 50% of cases. Aspirate of fluid from the abscess and its culture helps with the diagnosis. A CXR and abdominal ultrasound should be arranged. Amoebic serology should also be performed, which is positive in 90–95% of cases.

Radiology
On CXR, elevation of the right dome of the diaphragm, small pleural effusion or basal atelectasis may be seen. Ultrasound is a useful initial investigation and is sensitive in 80–90% of patients. Hypoechoic lesions with irregular outline may be seen. The abscesses may be multiple when the source is from the biliary tree. The CT scan is most useful in detection and evaluation of the abscesses. Contrast-enhanced CT shows well-defined hypodense lesions and they enhance peripherally. The CT may also help to identify any other co-existing intraabdominal pathology that may be a primary source.

Treatment
Antibiotics alone are not usually sufficient to treat liver abscesses. A combination of antibiotics and drainage of the abscess is the best option. Broad-spectrum antibiotics should be started and a close co-operation with the microbiologists is very important. Ultrasound or CT-guided aspiration may be performed but percutaneous catheter drainage is preferred. When there is failure to respond to the above-mentioned measures, open surgery may be needed.

Complications of liver abscess

- Empyema
- Rupture of the abscess into the peritoneal or pleural cavity
- Metastatic abscesses to other organs like lung, brain
- Septicaemia

2.14 B
2.15 A

Budd–Chiari syndrome

Budd–Chiari syndrome is a rare disorder and occurs due to obstruction in the hepatic venous outflow. The obstruction can be thrombotic or non-thrombotic. The exact prevalence is not known and as the condition is uncommon there is often a delay in the diagnosis. The obstruction to the blood flow leads to hepatic congestion and to liver cell injury, hepatic failure and portal hypertension. It is more common in women than men and the highest incidence is seen in the third or fourth decades of life.

Causes

1. *Haematological*:
   - Myeloproliferative disorders like polycythaemia vera
   - Paroxysmal nocturnal haemoglobinuria
   - Antiphospholipid syndrome
2. *Inherited conditions*:
   - Protein C & S deficiency
   - Factor V Leiden deficiency
   - Antithrombin III deficiency
3. Others:
   - Oral contraceptives, pregnancy, inflammatory bowel disease, intra-abdominal sepsis/abscesses, membranous webs, malignancy

Clinical features

A high index of suspicion is required to diagnose the condition. The classical triad is ascites, hepatomegaly and abdominal pain but they may not be always present and the symptoms may be non-specific. The onset may be acute but the presentation may also be subacute or chronic:

1. *Acute fulminant type*: it is uncommon and usually signifies severe underlying haematological disorder. There is jaundice, ascites, tender hepatomegaly and renal failure.
2. *Subacute type*: it may develop over a period of weeks and there is right hypochondrium pain and ascites. Hepatomegaly may be present but there are no stigmata of chronic liver disease.
3. *Chronic type*: this is the most common type. Jaundice may be absent but there may be hepatomegaly, ascites and other stigmata of chronic liver disease.

Diagnosis

The aim should be to determine if there is mechanical outflow obstruction, to find out any ongoing or established hepatic damage and to identify any underlying aetiological factor, e.g. haematological disorder.

Blood tests should include full blood count with platelets, U&Es, glucose, LFTs, albumin and coagulation screen. Ascitic fluid analysis should be carried out, which may show a protein level of 1.5–3.0 and serum-ascites albumin gradient > 1.1 g/dL; the WCC is usually < 100. Full haematological evaluation including a thrombophilia screen should be carried out. An ultrasound scan with Doppler flow studies should be carried out and CT or MRI is required for further evaluation. Hepatic venography is the gold standard test. Diagnosis is mainly by radiological imaging and liver biopsy.

Radiology

Ultrasound with Doppler flow studies is very sensitive and should be the initial radiological investigation. It can show absent blood flow in the hepatic vein or the flow may be reversed and it may show the thrombus.

The contrast-enhanced CT scan shows patchy enhancement of the liver tissue and post-hepatic IVC may be absent. The caudate lobe of the liver is usually enlarged and pre-hepatic dilatation of the IVC is seen but thrombus can be demonstrated in less than half of patients. Ascites and an enlarged spleen may be seen. The role of MRI in diagnosis of Budd–Chiari syndrome is still emerging. It can detect the blood flow or its absence in the hepatic vein or IVC.

Hepatic vein venography may help identify the thrombus and it may demonstrate a web as a cause of the obstruction. It also shows intrahepatic collaterals.

Differential diagnosis

- Metastatic disease
- Alcoholic liver disease
- Right-sided heart failure
- Granulomatous liver disease

Treatment

- *Medical:* This includes management of ascites, anticoagulation, antithrombotic therapy/angioplasty. The TIPS procedure may be required for subacute or chronic disease. For any underlying blood dyscrasias advice should be sought from the haematologists.
- *Surgical:* This is in the form of shunt operations or liver transplantation.

2.16 A
2.17 C

Renal cell carcinoma

Renal cell carcinoma (RCC) is the most common primary kidney malignancy, accounting for 90–95%. It usually arises from the epithelial cells of the proximal tubule. It may be resistant to chemotherapy or radiotherapy but may be responsive to newer biological agents like interferon-α (IFN-α).

Risk factors

- Cigarette smoking (strong relationship)
- Obesity
- Von Hippel-Lindau syndrome
- Renal dialysis
- Adult polycystic kidney disease
- Tuberous sclerosis
- Post renal transplant patients on immunosuppressants

Clinical features

The symptoms may be non-specific and hence the diagnosis may be delayed. Frank or occult haematuria may be the presenting feature. The classical triad of loin pain, haematuria and abdominal or flank mass is seen only in 10–20% of individuals. The patients may present with weight loss, anorexia, anaemia, night sweats and hypertension. Anaemia is a sign of advanced disease. Varicocele that is left sided may be present. It may also present as PUO. RCC can metastasize to the lungs (the most common site), liver, lymph nodes and bones, and resolution of the metastatic lesions and blood abnormalities may be seen with treatment.

Some paraneoplastic syndromes associated with RCC are:

- Erythrocytosis
- *Stauffer syndrome*: hepatic dysfunction without metastatic disease, which is reversible with resection of the tumour
- Hypercalcaemia
- Acquired dysfibrinogenaemia

Diagnosis

The initial blood tests should include complete blood count, ESR, U&Es, LFTs, calcium profile and coagulation screen. Urine analysis should be performed. Radiological investigations like ultrasound, CXR, CT or MRI are required for diagnosis and further characterization.

Radiology

On ultrasound, RCC can appear hyperechoic or hypoechoic. It is less sensitive than CT or MRI in staging of the tumour. It can be useful in evaluation of cystic lesions. CT is the investigation of choice for detection and staging of RCC. On non-contrast CT the tumour appears heterogeneous and on contrast enhancement it enhances non-homogeneously. It also shows associated calcification in the renal parenchyma. It provides important information on extrarenal extension, blood vessel invasion and lymph node involvement. On MRI, it appears hyopintense on T1-weighted images and hyperintense on T2-weighted images. It enhances heterogeneously with gadolinium.

Treatment

The localized disease is treated with radical nephrectomy. Following surgery adjuvant treatment like chemotherapy or radiotherapy does not improve the outcome. If metastases are present surgery has no role except in the case of haemorrhage or pain. Biological agents like IFN-α and IL-1 may produce tumour regression in 10–20% of patients but the results are not consistent.

Obstructive jaundice

Obstructive jaundice occurs due to blockage in the flow of bile. It can be extrahepatic (80% of cases) or intrahepatic (20%). In most cases it occurs secondary to choledocholithiasis when a stone causes obstruction in the common bile duct.

Causes

1. *Extrahepatic*:
   - CBD stone
   - Pancreatic carcinoma or carcinoma of ampulla of Vater
   - CBD stricture
   - Cholangiocarcinoma
   - Portal lymphadenopathy
   - Choledochal cyst

2. *Intrahepatic*:
   - Hepatocellular diseases: drugs (e.g. chlorpromazine, augmentin [amoxicillin and clavulanic acid], anabolic steroids), viral hepatitis, alcoholic hepatitis, TPN
   - Primary biliary cirrhosis (PBC)
   - Primary sclerosing cholangitis (PSC)

Clinical features
The initial complaint may be of pruritus and is followed by jaundice. Other features include malaise, anorexia, biliary colic, pale stools and dark urine. If the patients have fever, chills and rigors, cholangitis should be suspected. A carcinoma of the head of the pancreas may manifest as painless jaundice. Scratch marks from itching and xanthelesma may be a feature of PBC. When the gallbladder is palpable it usually means obstruction of the CBD due to a malignancy, e.g. carcinoma of the head of the pancreas as opposed to obstruction due to stone disease, in which case the gallbladder is not palpable (Courvoisier's law). In longstanding biliary obstruction deficiency of fat-soluble vitamins A, D, E and K may be seen. Prolonged obstruction to the bile flow also leads to secondary biliary cirrhosis, which may progress in spite of removing the obstruction.

Diagnosis
The investigations should be directed to confirm the diagnosis and to find the underlying cause. In all cases FBC, LFTs, U&Es, glucose, CRP/ESR and clotting screen should be done. A cholestatic pattern of abnormality on LFTs may be seen (i.e. ALP > ALT). A serum bilirubin level > 350 μmol/L may be seen in malignant obstruction. The ALP may be elevated 3–10 times higher than normal and the raised ALP may precede the onset of jaundice. GGT is also usually elevated. When obstruction is relieved, ALT is first to settle followed by serum bilirubin, which may take 2–3 weeks. The ALP levels fall very slowly and usually lag behind bilirubin levels.

Ultrasound should be the initial radiological investigation in the evaluation of cholestatic jaundice. Other investigations like CT scan, MRCP or ERCP may be required. ERCP may also prove to be therapeutic. Non-invasive tests like MRCP are preferable in evaluation as compared to the invasive techniques like ERCP.

Radiology

- *Ultrasound*: it is a good initial radiological investigation. It can show a dilated CBD or intrahepatic bile ducts but it may fail to show stones in the CBD. It can help differentiate between intrahepatic and extrahepatic causes. The gallbladder can be evaluated and the stones in the gallbladder may be identified.
- *CT scan*: with CT scan the hepatobiliary anatomy can be better visualized and the level of obstruction can be determined. However it may not always identify CBD stones as many of them may be radiolucent.
- *MRCP*: it is a non-invasive and very sensitive tool in the investigation of cholestatic jaundice. It provides excellent delineation of the biliary tree and pancreatic duct. It can help identify dilatation of the bile ducts, CBD stones and strictures. It can help diagnose malignant lesions and when combined with MRI the surrounding structures can also be evaluated.
- *PTC*: it is indicated when ERCP has failed or is contraindicated. This is very helpful in evaluation of dilated bile ducts and pancreatography can also be performed at the same time. The added advantage is that biliary or pancreatic cytology can be sent and percutaneous transhepatic drainage can be performed.

Treatment

After the diagnosis is made the aim should be the relief of the biliary obstruction. Broad-spectrum intravenous antibiotics are required if there is any suspicion of cholangitis.

2.20 C
2.21 B

Acute pancreatitis

Pancreatitis is inflammation of the pancreas and can be divided into acute and chronic types. Acute pancreatitis can range from a mild type to a severe form called 'necrotizing type', which has widespread systemic manifestations and carries a high rate of mortality.

Causes

- Gallstones
- Alcoholism
- Hyperlipidaemia
- Trauma
- Postoperative
- Drugs like azathioprine, tetracycline, sulphonamides, steroids
- Iatrogenic (secondary to ERCP)
- Carcinoma of the pancreas

Clinical features

The main symptom is abdominal pain, which can be mild to severe. It is boring in type and gets worse on lying supine. There may be associated nausea, vomiting and fever. There may be evidence of haemodynamic instability in the presence of shock. The patients may be tachypnoeic. A purple discoloration of the flanks may occur (Turner's sign) or there may be discoloration around the umbilicus (Cullen's sign); these may be indicative of necrotizing pancreatitis, which carries a poor prognosis. There may be guarding or rigidity. Later, a pancreatic pseudocyst may be palpable. A pleural effusion may develop, which is usually left sided.

Factors associated with poor outcome are:

- Hypotension (systolic BP less than 90 mmHg)
- Hypoxemia
- Renal impairment
- High CRP
- High WCC
- Haematocrit > 44%
- High glucose levels (>10 mmol/L)
- Hypocalcaemia (< 2 mmol/L)
- Serum albumin of < 32 g/L

Diagnosis

A raised white cell count is commonly seen. Serum amylase is raised usually more than 1000 u/mL but more than three times normal favour the diagnosis of pancreatitis. It should be borne in mind that raised serum amylase may be seen in many other clinical conditions and serum lipase or trypsin levels may resolve this dilemma. The PCV may be elevated to more than 50% and hyperglycaemia may be present. Hypoglycaemia is seen in about 25% of patients. LFTs may be deranged. LDH should be checked and high levels imply a poor prognosis. Other findings include raised triglyceride levels and hypoalbuminaemia, which indicates a poor prognosis. Radiological investigations like ultrasound or CT scan help to confirm the diagnosis.

Radiology

An AXR should be obtained to rule out a perforated bowel when presentation is acute. An ultrasound of the abdomen is a good initial radiological investigation, though it has its limitations as the pancreatitis may be missed in about 15–20% cases; it can however show the presence of gallstones.

CT scan helps to confirm the diagnosis but it may not be necessary to do it on presentation as the radiological findings may take 48–72 hours after onset of symptoms. It can be helpful when diagnosis is not clear and it can be very helpful to detect complications. MRCP can be helpful to identify any biliary or pancreatic duct obstruction in the presence of acute pancreatitis.

Differential diagnosis

- Perforated abdominal viscus
- Myocardial infarction

- Aortic dissection
- Pneumonia
- Acute cholecystitis

Complications

- *Pancreatic pseudocyst* (usually develops 1–4 weeks after onset of symptoms), abscess and haemorrhage, ARDS, shock, pericardial effusion, DIC, GI haemorrhage, portal vein thrombosis.
- *Rare:* Purtscher's retinopathy – sudden loss of vision is seen and there may be cotton wool spots and haemorrhages on fundoscopy. It occurs due to occlusion of posterior retinal artery by aggregated leucocytes.

Section 3: Central Nervous System

Questions

3.1 A 68-year-old man presented with left-sided hemiparesis, aphasia and gaze abnormalities. A CT scan carried out 24 hours after the onset of symptoms is shown. What is your diagnosis?

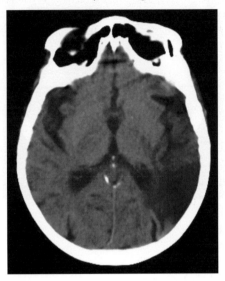

    A. MCA infarct
    B. Posterior cerebral artery infarct
    C. Lacunar infarct
    D. Anterior cerebral artery infarct

3.2 What should be the initial radiological investigation?

    A. A contrast-enhanced CT of the head
    B. MRI of the head
    C. Non-contrast CT of the head
    D. MR diffusion imaging

3.3 Choose the correct response:

    A. In acute ischaemic stroke, blood pressure should be treated when diastolic BP is > 90 mmHg.
    B. Thrombolysis with alteplase may be given within up to 6 hours of onset of symptoms.
    C. There is no relationship between the size of infarct in MCA territory and overall mortality.
    D. The earliest CT sign is increased attenuation of the MCA (dense MCA sign).

3.4 A 62-year-old man presented with headache, left-sided hemiparesis, vomiting and reduced level of consciousness. An urgent CT scan of the head was carried out and is shown. What is the diagnosis?

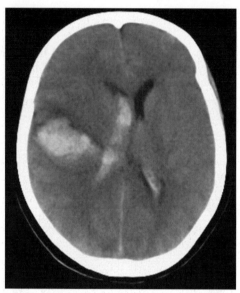

A. Meningioma
B. Cerebral abscess
C. Cerebral infarction
D. Intracerebral haemorrhage

3.5 Choose the correct response:

A. Haemoglobin concentration may affect the CT density of the haemorrhage.
B. Overall prognosis is not affected by the presence of blood in the ventricular system.
C. MRI is the preferred initial investigation in suspected intracranial haemorrhage.
D. Surrounding oedema is seen on the CT scan within first few hours.

3.6 All the following are true except:

A. The most common site of hypertensive intracerebral haemorrhage is putamen and internal capsule.
B. Cerebral amyloid angiopathy is associated with systemic amyloidosis.
C. Cocaine abuse can cause both haemorrhagic and ischaemic stroke.
D. Evacuation of the cerebral haematoma is usually not possible.

3.7 A 56-year-old woman presented with an episode of collapse, severe headache, nausea and photophobia. A CT scan was carried out and is shown. What is the most likely diagnosis?

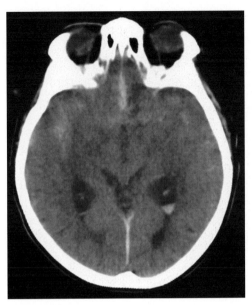

A. Meningitis
B. Cerebral venous thrombosis
C. Subarachnoid haemorrhage (SAH)
D. Intracerebral haemorrhage

3.8 The sensitivity of non-contrast CT scan in detecting subarachnoid haemorrhage in the first 24 hours is in the order of:

A. 90%
B. 70%
C. 60%
D. 50%

3.9 All the following are true except:

A. 70% of cases of SAHs are due to a Berry aneurysm.
B. Hypomagnesaemia in SAH is associated with a poor outcome.
C. SAH can be safely ruled out if CT scan is negative for SAH 3 weeks or more after the onset of symptoms.
D. Non-contrast CT is preferred to MRI scan as the initial investigation in suspected SAH.

3.10 A 45-year-old man presents with occipital headache, fever and vertigo. An MRI of the head was carried out and is shown. What is the most likely diagnosis?

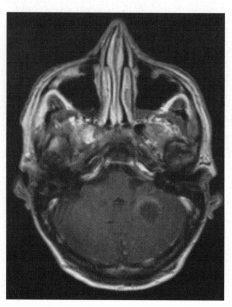

A. Cerebellar haemorrhage
B. Cerebellar abscess
C. Cerebellopontine angle tumour
D. Cerebellar infarction

3.11 All the following are true for cerebellar abscess except:

A. Hydrocephalus can occur.
B. It can occur in immunodefiency states like HIV.
C. The haematogenous route is the most common route of infection.
D. A CXR is a essential.

3.12 A 30-year-old woman presented with complaints of blurring of vision, fatigue, gait disturbance and paraesthesiae in hands of 2-days' duration. An MRI scan of the head was carried out and is shown. All the following may be seen in the CSF of this patient except:

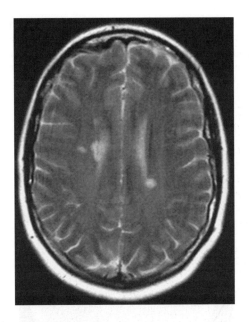

A. Mononuclear cell pleocytosis
B. Raised intrathecally synthesized IgG
C. Normal or mildly elevated proteins
D. High polymorphonuclear leucocytes

3.13 All the following are true of MS except:

A. Contrast-enhanced MRI can usually distinguish between old and acute MS plaques.
B. There is strong correlation between the number of lesions on the MRI and the neurological abnormalities.
C. The plaques are well circumscribed on MRI.
D. The plaques are seen in white matter close to the ventricles.

3.14 Choose the correct response:

A. Exercise-induced fatigue is not a feature of MS.
B. Methylprednisolone helps to prevent recurrences of MS.
C. Serum protein electrophoresis should be done before starting β-interferon therapy.
D. Cold temperatures may exacerbate MS symptoms.

3.15 A 65-year-old man presented with headache, mild confusion and unsteadiness on walking. His past medical history consists of atrial fibrillation, for which he takes warfarin. An urgent CT scan of the head was carried out, which is shown. What is the most likely diagnosis?

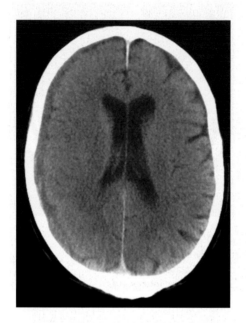

A. Epidural haematoma
B. Intracerebral haemorrhage
C. Acute subdural haematoma
D. Chronic subdural haematoma

3.16 Choose the correct answer:

A. MRI is more sensitive than CT to detect SDH.
B. The epidural haematoma has a concave inner margin but convex outer margin.
C. The CT density of the acute SDH persists even after 3 weeks.
D. The SDH is seen limited by the suture lines in the skull.

3.17 A 40-year-old woman presented with symptoms of headache, double vision and vomiting. She is known to have ulcerative colitis. The patient initially had a CT and then an MR angiography. The images are shown. Which of the following may be helpful in the treatment?

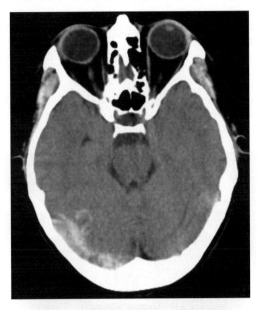

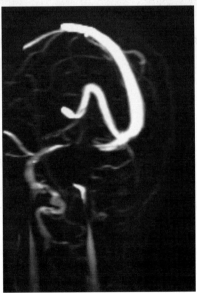

A. Antibiotics
B. Craniotomy and evacuation of haematoma
C. Anticoagulants
D. High-dose steroids

3.18 Choose the most appropriate response:

A. The diagnosis of cerebral venous sinus thrombosis is best established by MRA.
B. Lateral sinus is most commonly involved in cerebral venous sinus thrombosis.
C. The distribution of the venous infarct closely follows the arterial territories.
D. Haemorrhage is never a presenting feature of dural sinus thrombosis.

3.19 A 45-year-old man presented with headache, lethargy, loss of libido and visual disturbances. A CT scan was carried out and is shown. Choose the correct response in relation to the image shown:

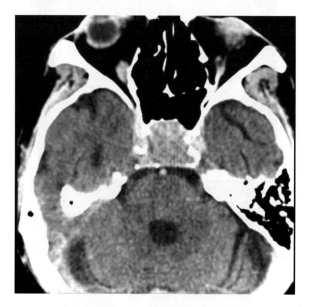

A. Headache is invariably seen in this type of tumour.
B. On plain skull X-ray, the enlargement of the pituitary fossa is symmetrical.
C. The initial diagnosis can be confidently made with CT scan.
D. Hypoprolectinemia is an associated feature.

3.20 All of the following are features of MEN 1 syndrome except:

A. Parathyroid adenomas
B. Pancreatic adenomas
C. Pituitary adenoma
D. Medullary carcinoma of the thyroid

3.21 All the following are true regarding pituitary tumours except:

A. Microadenomas can be diagnosed on MRI.
B. Pituitary tumours constitute 10% of all intracranial tumours.
C. They are a feature of McCune–Albright syndrome.
D. Thyroid stimulating hormone-secreting tumours are very common.

3.22 A 72-year-old man presented with confusion, vomiting and seizures. A CT scan is shown, which shows the presence of cerebral metastases. The least likely site of primary tumour is:

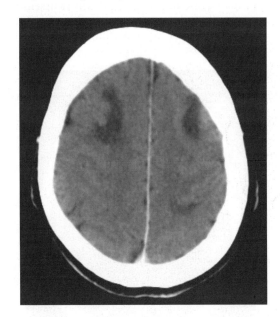

A. Colon
B. Prostate
C. Melanoma
D. Thyroid

3.23 The imaging modality of choice in suspected brain metastases is:

A. Contrast-enhanced CT
B. Non-contrast CT
C. Diffusion-weighted MR
D. Contrast-enhanced MR

3.24 All the following are true except:

A. A lesion that does not enhance on contrast enhancement is unlikely to be a metastatic lesion.
B. It is rare for ovarian cancer to metastasize to the brain.
C. Colonic carcinoma is the commonest primary causing cerebral metastasis.
D. If a single brain metastasis is seen on CT, co-existent metastatic lesions should be excluded with contrast-enhanced MRI.

3.25 A 70-year-old man presented with gradually worsening headache of 5 weeks' duration with daily vomiting on waking up in the morning and unsteadiness of gait. A CT scan of the head was carried out and is shown. What is the most likely diagnosis?

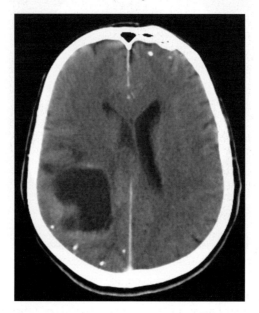

A. Encephalitis
B. Glioblastoma multiforme
C. Acoustic neuroma
D. Intracerebral haemorrhage

3.26 Choose the correct response:

A. Amongst astrocytomas, glioblastoma multiforme, seen in older age groups, carries the worst prognosis.
B. CNS lymphoma in HIV has a better prognosis than systemic lymphoma.
C. Ependymomas carry a very poor prognosis.
D. Calcification is never a feature of astrocytomas.

3.27 A 50-year-old woman presented with features of headache, seizures, psychosis and parkinsonian features. Her past medical history consisted of treatment for Hodgkin's lymphoma. An MRI scan of the head was carried out and is shown. What is the most likely diagnosis?

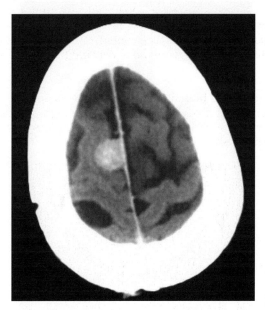

A. Glioblastoma multiforme
B. Parasagittal meningioma
C. Craniopharyngioma
D. Brain metastases

3.28 All the following are true regarding meningioma except:

A. A dural tail on CT is pathognomonic of meningioma.
B. Anosmia is a feature of olfactory groove meningioma.
C. Multiple cranial nerve palsies may be a feature of sphenoid ridge meningioma.
D. Hyperostosis of the adjacent skull is seen.

3.29 All of the following are a feature of Kennedy–Foster syndrome:

A. Ipsilateral optic atrophy
B. Contralateral optic atrophy
C. Anosmia
D. Contralateral papilloedema

3.30 A 66-year-old patient presented with occipital headache, unsteadiness of gait and vomiting. An urgent CT of the head was carried out and is shown. What is the diagnosis?

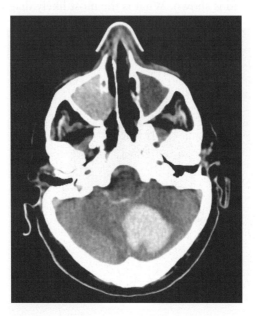

A. Central pontine myelinolysis
B. Cerebellar haemorrhage
C. Posterior cerebral artery stroke
D. Intracerebral haemorrhage

3.31 Choose the correct response in relation to cerebellar haemorrhage:

A. Altered level of consciousness is common at presentation.
B. Brainstem herniation is very uncommon.
C. The hydrocephalus is usually of obstructive type.
D. Small and laterally located haematomas with no signs of clinical progression can be conservatively managed.

3.32 A 68-year-old man presented with leg weakness, urinary retention and a history of weight loss. An MRI of the spine was carried out and is shown. All the following may be true except:

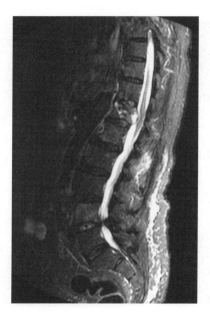

A. High-dose dexamethasone should be started.
B. Radiotherapy may be required.
C. Involvement of the sphincter does not affect the outcome.
D. Extensor plantar reflex denotes significant cord compression.

3.33 Choose the correct response:

A. Prostatic metastases commonly metastasize to the thoracic spine.
B. Intact sensation over the sacral region (sacral sparing) is seen in intramedullary tumours.
C. Sphincter disturbance is very common with cauda equina syndrome.
D. The intervertebral disc is not involved in infection.

3.34 A 45-year-old man presented with headache, fever and reduced consciousness levels. A CT scan of the head was carried out and is shown. What is the most likely diagnosis?

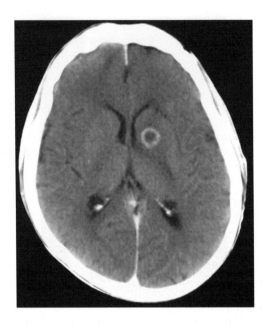

A. Cerebritis
B. Encephalitis
C. Subdural empyema
D. Brain abscess

3.35 In case of haematogenous spread, the brain abscess is usually seen in:

A. MCA territory
B. Posterior cerebral artery territory
C. Anterior cerebral artery territory
D. Cerebellum

3.36 All the following are true except:

A. Fever is invariably present in brain abscess.
B. Multiple abscesses may be seen in HIV patients.
C. When abscess is seen in the temporal lobe, otogenic infection as a cause should be suspected.
D. MRI is more sensitive in detecting brain abscess than CT scan.

Answers

3.1 A
3.2 C
3.3 D

Stroke

Stroke is a major cause of disability. It consists of group of disorders where sudden loss of cerebral blood flow to an area of the brain causes neurological deficit lasting more than 24 hours.

Subtypes of stroke:

1. Ischaemic (80%)
    A. *Thrombotic*: from within intracerebral arteries, ulcerated plaque at carotid artery bifurcation, prothrombotic states like sickle cell anaemia, protein C deficiency and polycythaemia
    B. *Embolic*: from extracranial arteries or from heart, e.g. atrial fibrillation, prosthetic heart valves, endocarditis
2. Haemorrhagic
3. Subarachnoid haemorrhage
4. In young persons, substance misuse, vasculitis and carotid artery dissection should be suspected

Risk factors

1. Advancing age
2. Smoking
3. Coronary artery disease
4. Hypertension
5. Hypercholesterolaemia
6. Atrial fibrillation

Clinical features

The signs and symptoms depend on the area of brain affected. They may be a combination of monoparesis, hemiparesis, aphasia, dysarthria, visual field defects and ataxia.

The stroke syndromes:

1. Middle cerebral artery (MCA) syndrome
2. Anterior cerebral artery syndrome
3. Posterior cerebral artery syndrome
4. Lacunar infarcts
5. Vertebrobasilar

The Oxfordshire Community Stroke Project (OCSP) is used to classify the clinical syndromes and if the infarct is not seen on the CT it can be used to predict the site.

The OCSP classification:

1. Total anterior circulation (TAC): combination of 'three of three' of:
   • Weakness (with/without sensory deficit) of at least two of three body areas (face/arm/leg)
   • Homonymous hemianopia
   • Higher cerebral dysfunction (dysphasia, dyspraxia commonest). If the patient is drowsy with unilateral weakness, the last two factors are assumed.
2. Partial anterior circulation (PAC)
   • Two of three of TAC criteria or restricted motor/sensory deficit, e.g. one limb, face and hand or higher cerebral dysfunction alone
   • More restricted cortical infarcts – occlusion of branches of MCA (e.g. upper division – usually no field defect; lower – motor/sensory defect negligible)
3. Lacunar (LAC)
   • Pure motor (most common). Complete or incomplete weakness of one side, involving the whole of two of three body areas (face/arm/leg). Sensory symptoms, dysarthria or dysphasia allowed
   • Pure sensory. Sensory symptoms and/or signs, same distribution
   • Sensorimotor. Combination of the above
   • Ataxic hemiparesis. Hemiparesis and ipsilateral cerebral ataxia
4. Posterior circulation (POC)
   • Affecting brainstem, cerebral or occipital lobes

Diagnosis
All patients should have a full blood count, U&E, glucose, lipids and coagulation screen carried out. An ECG should be obtained.

Radiology
A non-contrast CT head should be obtained initially. This helps in distinguishing haemorrhagic from non-haemorrhagic stroke. This also rules out other conditions like a space-occupying lesion, abscess, metastases or a haematoma. CT is most sensitive when carried out after 24 h of the onset of symptoms. When the initial scan is equivocal it should be repeated after 48 hours. An infarct area is seen in 80% of patients. A large infarct size (> 50%) in the MCA territory carries increased mortality.

The earliest CT sign is increased attenuation of the MCA (dense MCA sign) and it carries a poor prognosis. The other signs of ischaemia that may be seen are loss of differentiation between cortex and subcortical white matter, obscuration of lentiform nucleus and effacement of cerebral sulci.

The imaging in acute stroke is developing at a rapid pace and nowadays there is emphasis on early detection of the infarct. MRI is proving to be helpful and MR diffusion imaging is more sensitive in detecting early parenchymal changes. This may be useful in selecting patients likely to fit the criteria for thrombolysis.

Treatment
• Complete evaluation is needed but the patient should be stabilized first with particular attention to the airway support.

- Blood pressure and blood glucose should be monitored.
- Intracranial pressure (ICP) monitoring may be required and also ways to reduce raised ICP may be needed.
- Supportive care – to look for and treat fever, hyperglycaemia, dehydration and hypoxia
- Secondary prophylaxis and risk factor modification
- Rehabilitation
- *Medical management*: this consists of anti-platelet agents, anti-coagulants and thrombolysis. The thrombolytic agent used is alteplase. This is helpful in carefully selected patients and is available only in specialist centres. It should be administered < 3 hours from the acute event and when contra-indications are ruled out.

Differential diagnosis (stroke mimics)

- Trauma
- Meningitis/encephalitis
- Cerebral neoplasm
- Post ictal state
- *Metabolic*: hyponatremic, hyperosmolar non-ketotic coma, hypoglycaemia

3.4 D
3.5 A
3.6 B

Intracerebral haemorrhage

Intracrebral haemorrhage is most common type of intracranial haemorrhage. It accounts for 10% of all strokes and carries higher mortality rate than ischaemic strokes.

Risk factors

- Hypertension
- Advanced age
- Alcoholism
- Anticoagulation
- Cerebral amyloid angiopathy
- Cocaine abuse

Clinical features
It occurs usually during the daytime when the patient is awake during stress. The usual symptoms are a reduced level of consciousness, headache, seizures, and dysarthria and in the later stages stupor and coma. Putamen is the most common site and usually the internal capsule also gets involved and hence contralateral hemiplegia/hemiparesis is present. Usually it develops over a period of 30–90 minutes but the duration may be longer in patients taking anticoagulants. It is difficult to distinguish haemorrhagic from ischaemic stroke clinically but symptoms like headache, vomiting, reduced level of consciousness and hypertension are seen more commonly with haemorrhagic stroke.

- *Hypertensive haemorrhage*: this occurs due to rupture of small penetrating arteries deep in the brain and the common sites are basal ganglia, cerebellum and pons. When haemorrhage occurs in other areas of the brain or in normotensive individuals, other disorders like blood dyscrasias or arteriovenous malformations should be suspected. Blood may enter the ventricular system and cause hydrocephalus.
- *Thalamic haemorrhage*: contralateral hemiplegia, sensory deficit, aphasia and various eye signs may be present.
- *Pontine haemorrhage*: quadriplegia, pin-point pupils, coma along with doll's eye movements may be seen.
- *Cerebellar haemorrhage*: this is discussed in detail in section 3.12.
- *Cerebral amyloid angiopathy*: this occurs in the elderly and is due to arteriolar degeneration, which leads to deposition of amyloid in the walls of the cerebral arteries and causes multifocal lobar haemorrhages. It is also associated with haemorrhage following thrombolysis for acute myocardial infarction. It is not associated with systemic amyloidosis.
- *Cocaine abuse*: it may cause ischaemic stroke, intracerebral or subarachnoid haemorrhage. It causes stroke in young people and is probably due to hypertension produced by cocaine.

Diagnosis
All patients should have a full blood count, U&E, glucose, lipids, coagulation screen and an ECG.

Radiology
A CT scan of the head helps to differentiate between haemorrhagic and non-haemorrhagic stroke. A non-contrast CT of the head should be obtained initially and it detects haemorrhage in the supratentorial space, which appears as increased radiographic density. With contrast-enhanced CT, a cerebral tumour may appear to be of same density as the haemorrhage. The CT density of the haemorrhage is determined by the haemoglobin concentration and the extracellular fluid.

Initially, there is no surrounding oedema and the bleeding appears as a homogeneous density. When the clot retracts a thin rim is seen. Blood is seen in the ventricles when bleeding is extensive and may appear as fluid level. At later stages a contrast-enhanced CT shows an area of enhancement due to vasogenic oedema. After many weeks the density of the blood products may appear similar to that of brain or CSF.

The MRI findings of intracerebral haemorrhage follow a time course due to presence of haemoglobin and its degradation products. A CT scan should be the preferred investigation for intracerebral haemorrhage.

Treatment
This condition carries a high rate of mortality, which depends on the size and location of the haematoma; the presence of blood in the ventricles worsens the prognosis. Usually evacuation of the haematoma is possible in cerebellar haemorrhage but not in cerebral haemorrhage. When there is evidence of raised intracranial pressure osmotic agents like mannitol and induced hyperventilation may be helpful. With good, supportive care recovery may be good as the surrounding brain tissue is compressed but not infarcted.

3.7 C
3.8 A
3.9 C

Subarachnoid haemorrhage

Subarachnoid haemorrhage (SAH) accounts for 5% of all strokes. The most common cause is rupture of a Berry aneurysm. Outcome is determined by the degree of the neurological deficit. Half of the patients die and one-third are left with a disability.

Causes

- Saccular or Berry aneurysm (70%)
- Arteriovenous malformation (10%)
- Hypertension (10%)
- Idiopathic (5%)

Berry aneurysm: It is found on autopsy in about 8% of individuals. They are asymptomatic but it can cause sudden death. The usual location is arterial bifurcations; the common sites are posterior communication artery in 30%, anterior communication in 25% and middle cerebral artery in 25%.

Clinical features

The classical history is of sudden, severe headache that peaks in minutes and the patients describe it to be the worst pain they've experienced in their life. Other symptoms are nausea, vomiting, photophobia, seizures, neck stiffness and reduced level of consciousness. There may be a history of loss of consciousness and signs of focal neurological deficit. Fundoscopy may reveal sub-hyaloid haemorrhages. Sometimes sentinel bleeds may occur associated with headache.

Diagnosis

Initial investigations: Blood tests including full blood count, coagulation screen, U&Es, serum glucose, serum magnesium and ECG. Hyponatremia may be present and also hypomagnesaemia, which is associated with a poor outcome.

An urgent CT scan of the head should be arranged and if it is negative then a lumbar puncture is required, which shows xanthochromia and raised CSF pressure. A CT angiography is required after the diagnosis is confirmed to identify the site of aneurysm.

If the CT scan and LP are negative within 2 weeks of onset of symptoms then an alternate diagnosis should be considered. The sensitivity of CT decreases after 10 days and xanthochromia is seen in 70% in 3 weeks and in 40% after 4 weeks and hence if a patient presents after 2 weeks and SAH is suspected, he or she should be referred to a neurosurgical unit for further evaluation.

Radiology

A non-contrast CT (NCCT) of the head has a sensitivity of 90% in the first 24 hours and this reduces to 50% by 72 hours. With time blood gets reabsorbed and the scan may appear to be normal. The bleed appears as increased density of CSF spaces. This density is dependent on the haemoglobin concentration. Blood is seen in the basal cisterns as most of the aneurysms are in close relation to the circle of Willis. Sometimes a small clot can be seen near the site of the rupture, which provides a clue to the origin.

NCCT should be the preferred investigation as compared to the MRI scan. The sensitivity of MRI increases with FLAIR sequence as compared to the conventional spin-echo sequence and the SAH appears as an area of high signal. A CT or MRI helps to identify complications like vasospasm-induced ischaemia and hydrocephalus.

Differential diagnosis

- Intracerebral haemorrhage
- Cerebral venous thrombosis
- Subdural haematoma
- Cluster headache
- Cerebral neoplasm
- Meningitis

Treatment

Early diagnosis and referral to a neurosurgical unit is important as early intervention can improve outcome.

Close monitoring is required to detect any worsening of Glasgow Coma Scale (GCS), cardiopulmonary dysfunction and signs of raised intracranial pressure. Particular attention should be given to the hydration status and to correct electrolyte abnormalities.

Nimodipine reduces the risk of poor outcome and delayed cerebral ischaemia. Definitive treatment is in the form of clipping of the aneurysm. The vasospasm is at its maximum at 5 days and the surgery is usually delayed up to 10 days after the bleed.

Patients should be advised to stop smoking; alcohol should be taken only in moderation and blood pressure monitored.

Outcome

The overall case–fatality rate is about 45%. More than 50% of survivors are left with disability. The risk of re-bleeding is 25% at 2 weeks, 40% at 4 weeks, 60% at 6 months and 3% per year thereafter. The factors that influence the prognosis adversely are impaired level of consciousness, increasing age and large volume of blood on CT.

Complications

- *Re-bleeding*
- *Ischaemic infarction secondary to vasospasm*: it may occur 4–11 days after SAH and is a significant cause of morbidity. The risk is increased when a significant amount of blood is present on the initial CT.
- *Hydrocephalus*: this is usually of the communicating type. It may develop within a few hours and may be seen as mild dilatation of the ventricles. Often it may resolve and if not a shunt procedure may be required.

3.10 B
3.11 C

Cerebellar abscess

Cerebellar abscess arises from either septic emboli or direct extension from infections like mastoiditis or secondary to trauma.

Causes

- Otogenic diseases like mastoiditis, sinusitis (most common mode of infection)
- Tuberculosis
- Immunocompromised states like HIV
- Septic embolus: endocarditis, lung infections like bronchiectasis, lung abscess
- Fungal

In the case of haematogenous infections multiple abscesses may be seen.

Clinical features

- Headache, usually suboccipital
- Nausea and vomiting
- Neck stiffness
- Pyrexia
- Dysdiadokinesia
- Nystagmus and vertigo

Diagnosis

The blood tests show high inflammatory markers. In all cases a CXR must be obtained.

A CT may show the abscess but an MRI is more helpful. With contrast ring enhancement surrounding oedema is seen.

Treatment

Treatment consists of surgical drainage with eradication of the primary focus of infection. Broad-spectrum antibiotics should be given. Patients should be monitored for the presence of any incipient hydrocephalus and appropriate management instituted as needed.

3.12 D
3.13 B
3.14 C

Multiple sclerosis

MS is a disease of young adults with possible autoimmune basis. There are disseminated patches of demyelination, often perivenular with reactive gliosis seen in the white matter of the brain and spinal cord. The episodes may be precipitated by an infection, trauma or after pregnancy.

Clinical features

There are multiple neurological deficits that may be characterized by remissions and relapses leading to disability. Exercise-induced weakness is characteristic. Excess heat in the form of a hot bath or warm weather may exacerbate the symptoms, most commonly paraesthesias in one or more limbs or the face, focal weakness, unsteadiness, visual disturbances like diplopia, partial loss of vision (retrobulbar neuritis), sphincter disturbances and spasticity in limbs. Optic neuritis and bilateral internuclear ophthalmoplegia are seen. Spinal cord involvement causes bladder dysfunction, e.g. urgency, hesitancy or incontinence. Erectile dysfunction in men may occur.

Types

- *Relapsing–remitting disease*: There is usually an interval of months or years between the initial episode and recurrence. Later, the interval between episodes may continue to decrease, leading to permanent disability.
- *Secondary progressive disease*: Sometimes progressive deterioration may occur unrelated to an acute event.
- *Primary progressive disease*: the symptoms continue to progress after onset, leading to early disability.

Diagnosis

- This is based on the presence of > 2 CNS, MRI, evoked potential and CSF abnormalities. Clinically, there should be a history of remitting and relapsing neurological symptoms and objective evidence of > 2 CNS abnormalities. The symptoms should be present for > 24 hours and two symptoms must have occurred at least 1 month apart.
- *CSF*: shows mononuclear cell pleocytosis and oligoclonal bands in the CSF.
- *Evoked potentials*: in 80–90% of patients with MS abnormalities in one or more evoked potential modalities (visual, auditory or somatosensory) is present.
- *Radiology*: MRI is the most sensitive imaging modality. Gadolinium-enhanced MRI can distinguish between an actively inflamed plaque and older plaques. The plaques are well circumscribed and there is no mass effect. They are seen in white matter close to the ventricles, which are mostly posterior. Acute lesions may be larger; however, the MS lesions on MRI may be asymptomatic and there is poor correlation between the number of lesions on MRI and the neurological abnormalities.

Differential diagnosis

- Anti-phospholipid syndrome
- Behçet's disease
- Systemic lupus
- Acute disseminated encephalitis
- Sarcoidosis

Treatment

The course of MS is very unpredictable. In general, treatment can be divided into treatment of acute attacks, treatment with disease-modifying agents and supportive treatment:

- Glucocorticoids (methylprednisolone) are used to treat first attacks or acute exacerbations. They reduce the severity and duration of attacks. It is important to rule out pseudo-exacerbations caused by hot temperature, fever or intercurrent infection. Plasma exchange may be helpful if patients are not responding to methylprednisolone.
- Disease-modifying agents like β-interferon or glatiramer acetate are used usually in relapsing–remitting and secondary progressive MS. The patients should fulfil the following criteria: ability to walk independently, at least two relapses over last 2 years, age 18 years or older and provided there are no contraindications. Contraindications to β-interferon therapy are severe depression and monoclonal gammopathy (protein electrophoresis should be carried out before starting therapy).
- Supportive treatment for spasticity, bladder dysfunction, pain, constipation, fatigue and depression helps to improve quality of life.

3.15 C
3.16 A

Subdural haematoma

SDH is haemorrhage beneath the dura and is the most common extra-axial collection. It may be life threatening as it causes mass effect on the adjacent brain tissue and can lead to a rise in intracranial pressure and brain herniation. It occurs due to bleeding from the bridging subdural veins, which connect the cerebral cortex to the dural sinuses.

It can be classified as:

- Hyperacute (< 12 hours)
- Acute (a few days)
- Subacute (a few days to 2–3 weeks)
- Chronic (> 3 weeks)

Clinical features
There is usually a history of injury. Often the patients may not be able to recall any injury, particularly the elderly and patients on oral anticoagulants or after decelerating injury. The onset of symptoms may be within minutes or hours but sometimes a lucid interval may be present.

There may be headache, mental changes, hemiparesis, stupor and coma. In the presence of raised intracranial pressure, there may be an ipsilateral dilated pupil and hemiparesis.

Diagnosis
CT of the head should be arranged on an urgent basis. The SDH appears crescent shaped with a concave inner and convex outer margin. There is usually midline shift. Dilatation of the contralateral ventricle is a bad prognostic sign. The density of haematoma on CT gradually decreases with time. It remains denser than brain for 1 week and is less dense after 3 weeks. On CT it is also important to look for evidence of brain contusion, skull fracture or subarachnoid bleed. MRI is more sensitive in detecting SDH than CT, but CT remains as the initial investigation of choice.

Differential diagnosis

- *Epidural haematoma*: This does not appear to be crescent shaped but rather convex on both inner and outer margins. The epidural haematoma does not cross the suture lines but may cross the midline.
- Arachnoid cyst

Treatment

- *Supportive treatment*: attention should be given to airway, breathing, circulation and the Glasgow Coma Scale.
- Patients should be monitored for any signs of raised intracranial pressure and appropriate measures taken like osmotic diuresis or hyperventilation.
- Definitive treatment is in the form of decompression surgery.

3.17 C
3.18 A

Central venous sinus thrombosis

Cerebral venous sinus thrombosis is an uncommon condition and it carries a high rate of mortality. It causes venous infarct secondary to thrombosis in the cerebral dural sinuses or in the cerebral veins. This can be multifocal and may present as haemorrhage. It is more common in women than men.

Causes

- Trauma and neurosurgical procedures like dural taps
- Infection of the paranasal sinuses
- Pregnancy and oral contraceptive use
- Inflammatory bowel disease
- Antiphospholipid syndrome, antithrombin 3 deficiency, lupus anticoagulant
- Sickle cell disease, polycythaemia
- Malignancy
- Systemic lupus erythematosus
- Nephrotic syndrome
- Dehydration

Clinical features
Headache may be the presenting feature. Nausea, vomiting, seizures, altered sensorium, visual field defects, cranial nerve palsies involving 3rd and 6th nerve, facial numbness and deafness may be present. If the thrombus extends into the jugular vein the patient may develop palsies of 9th, 10th, 11th and 12th nerves (jugular foramen syndrome). In cavernous sinus thrombosis, there may be ipsilateral periorbital oedema and proptosis, ptosis and facial numbness due to involvement of trigeminal nerve and extra-ocular muscle involvement. Superior sagittal sinus thrombosis is more common and may lead to unilateral lower limb weakness or paraplegia.

Diagnosis
Blood tests should be carried out to try to find the underlying cause: haemoglobin, white cell count, platelet counts, D-dimer, thrombophilia screen, Hb electrophoresis, LFTs, double-stranded DNA and ANCA. Urine should be checked for proteinuria.

Radiology
Imaging studies are helpful in establishing the diagnosis dural sinus thrombosis. A CT scan of the head should be carried out in the first instance. On CT, superior sagittal sinus thrombosis may appear as a bilateral parasagittal infarct. On contrast enhancement, the wall of the sinuses become hyperintense (delta sign). The distribution of the infarction may not correspond to the arterial distribution. The CT is also helpful to rule out intracranial tumours and subdural haematoma. If infection is suspected, a CT of the paranasal sinuses should also be included. MR, however, does not give any more benefit than CT. It shows absence of flow void in the dural sinuses. Phase-contrast MRA best demonstrates any occlusion in the dural sinus; it shows the flow but not the thrombus.

Differential diagnosis

- Subdural haematoma
- Pseudotumour cerebri
- Cerebral empyema
- Intracranial haemorrhage
- Cerebral metastases
- Head injury/brain contusion
- Vasculitic syndromes

Treatment

- *Supportive care*: attention should be given to airway and circulation, and hydration status. The GCS should be closely monitored. Anticonvulsants should be given to prevent seizures.
- *Specific treatment use of anticoagulant or thrombolytic therapy*: though there are varied views on anticoagulation as there is an increased risk of haemorrhage, thrombolytic therapy is used in specialized centres using the microcatheter technique.

3.19 C
3.20 D
3.21 D

Pituitary tumours

Pituitary tumours account for 10% of all intracranial tumours, and most of the tumours in the pituitary and suprasellar areas are adenomas. They are benign and slow growing and sometimes they may be discovered incidentally.

They arise in one of the five anterior pituitary cell types hence the clinical picture is dominated by the cell of origin of the tumour. They may be divided into functioning (secretory) or non-functioning (non-secretory) types. Tumours < 1 cm in size are called 'microadenomas'. They may also be classified by their staining characteristics. The large tumours can compress the adjacent anatomical structures like optic nerves.

Pituitary tumours may be associated with some genetic syndromes:

- *Multiple endocrine neoplasia (MEN 1)*: this is an autosomal dominant condition consisting of parathyroid, pancreatic and pituitary adenomas.
- *McCune–Albright syndrome*: this consists of skin pigmentation, polyostotic fibrous dysplasia, growth hormone secreting pituitary adenomas and adrenal adenomas.
- *Carney syndrome*: this consists of pituitary adenomas, skin pigmentation, myxomas and other endocrine tumours including testicular and adrenal adenomas.

Other suprasellar masses to be considered in conjunction with pituitary tumours are:

- Craniopharygiomas
- Histiocytosis X
- Meningioma
- Chordoma
- Pituitary metastases
- Rathke's cyst

Craniopharyngiomas arise in or near the pituitary stalk and are derived from the Rathke's pouch. They are cystic tumours and are locally invasive. The presentation is in the young, usually in the second decade and with signs of pressure effects like headache, vomiting, visual field defects and papilloedema. There may be cranial nerve palsies and mental changes. Diabetes insipidus may be seen along with anterior pituitary dysfunction. Affected children may present with growth retardation. Calcification is usually seen, which may be detected on the skull X-ray or on the CT. Treatment is usually trans-sphenoidal surgery with postoperative radiotherapy and pituitary hormone replacement.

Clinical features
Headache may be present and this is usually seen with macroadenomas. The headache is not related to the size of the tumour. The clinical presentation can be varied and can be divided into:

- *Hypopituitarism*: this is seen with macroadenomas and may manifest as hypogonadism, hypothyroidism, growth retardation, adrenal deficiency and hyperprolactinemia.
- *Hypersecretory tumours (causing hormonal excess)*: excess ACTH secretion leading to Cushing's disease, acromegaly secondary to growth hormone excess, prolactinoma and TSH-secreting tumours (rare).
- *Symptoms secondary to pressure effects*: these may cause neurological symptoms and are usually seen with macroadenomas. These include bitemporal hemianopia secondary to compression of the optic chiasm, scotomas

and reduced visual acuity, and the lateral growth may invade the cavernous sinus causing 3rd, 4th and 6th cranial nerve palsies.

Diagnosis
This should include a thorough neurological examination looking for papilloedema, visual field defects and other eye signs. In addition include hormonal tests to check for functioning pituitary adenomas and imaging.

The usual screening tests for secretory pituitary tumours include:

- *Acromegaly*: serum IGF-1 and oral glucose tolerance test with growth hormone
- *Cushing's disease*: ACTH assay, 24-hour urinary free cortisol levels and dexamethasone suppression test
- *Prolactinoma*: serum prolactin levels

Radiology
Though a diagnosis of macroadenoma can be made by CT, MRI is the investigation of choice for microadenomas. Most of the microadenomas become enhanced after contrast.

Macroadenomas: on plain X-ray, the pituitary fossa may appear asymmetrical and on a lateral view the 'double floor' sign may be seen. On CT scan, a soft tissue mass with density greater than brain is seen in an enlarged pituitary fossa. They usually enhance uniformly after the contrast, but if the enhancement is not uniform it may be due to necrosis within the tumour.

An assessment should be made for extrasellar extension as the tumours may invade the cavernous sinus, sphenoid sinus or the chiasmatic cistern. They may compress the optic chiasm or even hypothalamus. A radionuclide study like ^{111}In-octreotide scintigraphy is used to distinguish residual or recurrent tumours from postoperative scarring. It also identifies patients with macroadenoma likely to respond to octreotide therapy.

Empty sella syndrome: this term is used to denote an enlarged pituitary fossa that is filled with CSF. This is seen usually in the elderly and there may not be associated endocrine or neurological abnormalities. In younger patients this may be associated with benign intracranial hypertension.

Treatment
Trans-sphenoidal surgery is the preferred approach but it may not be possible with larger tumours, when a transfrontal approach may be required. The excised specimen should be sent for histological evaluation. Hypopituitarism is a complication.

For prolactinoma, dopaminergic receptor agonists like bromocriptine lead to marked symptomatic improvement including visual field abnormalities and other symptoms. Trans-sphenoidal surgery can also be curative. For acromegaly, somatostatin analogues are used. The surgical approach also helps reduce excess hormone secretion and symptoms secondary to mass effect. In Cushing's disease, this approach can be curative in more than 80% of patients. Radiotherapy can be used either as a primary treatment or as an adjunct to surgery.

3.22 B
3.23 D
3.24 C

Cerebral metastases

Metastases to the brain are the most feared complication of a cancer. They constitute 40% of intracranial tumours. They reach the brain mainly through the haematogenous route. Most of them are either from primary lung cancer or emboli from the pulmonary metastases. They are commonly multiple.

The cancers commonly leading to cerebral metastases are:

- Lung (commonest)
- Malignant melanoma
- Breast
- Renal cell carcinoma
- Colonic carcinoma
- Thyroid

Cerebral metastases with unknown primary are most likely from, in decreasing order, lung, breast, colon and melanoma.

Clinical features

The common symptoms are headache, nausea, vomiting (especially in the morning), confusion, seizures, visual field defects and focal weakness. Haemorrhage can occur in brain metastases leading to clinical deterioration.

Diagnosis

When primary cancer is known: in patients with known primary tumour when there are symptoms suggestive of brain metastases, an urgent contrast-enhanced CT scan of the head or an MRI should be arranged.

Radiology

Contrast enhancement increases the diagnostic accuracy of CT. Most of the metastases are located at the junction of white and grey mater and surrounding oedema is seen due to leaky blood vessels. 80% of these metastases are located in the cerebrum, about 15% in the cerebellum and 5% in the brainstem. If a solitary metastasis is seen, it is of utmost importance to rule out the presence of any other metastases within the brain as the management differs significantly for each condition.

MRI with contrast enhancement is the imaging modality of choice as it is more sensitive. Single or multiple well-demarcated lesions with surrounding oedema are seen. These lesions appear isointense and hyperintense on T1- and T2-weighted images, respectively. Exceptions are mucinous adenocarcinoma, which may be hypointense on T2, and haemorrhagic metastases or melanoma, which may appear hyperintense on T2-weighted images. Non-enhancing lesions following contrast enhancement are less likely to be metastatic lesions. Contrast-enhanced MRI also detects leptomeningeal involvement. Larger metastases appear as ring lesions with a central area of non-enhancement due to necrotic tissue as the tumour outgrows the blood supply.

Differential diagnosis

- Brain abscess
- Brain lymphoma
- Intracerebral haemorrhage
- Meningioma

Treatment

- The prognosis is very poor once cerebral metastases are detected. The aim should be palliative treatment to improve the quality of life and prolong survival, as it is incurable.
- *Supportive treatment*: glucocorticoids like dexamethasone are helpful in reducing the cerebral oedema and anticonvulsants like phenytoin should be used when there are seizures.
- Single metastatic lesion may be amenable to surgical removal, prolonging survival.
- Cerebral irradiation is a more specific treatment. Radiosurgery can be helpful when there are 2–3 but not 4 or more metastases.

Important points

- Breast carcinoma that metastasizes to bone does not metastasize to brain.
- Ductal breast carcinoma has a tendency to metastasize to the cerebellum and posterior pituitary.
- All tumours that metastasize to the lungs can metastasize to the brain.
- Tumours that rarely cause cerebral metastases are: ovary, prostate and Hodgkin's lymphoma.

Other causes of multiple brain lesions:

- Toxoplasmosis
- Lymphoma
- Cerebral abscesses
- Multicentric glioma

Other causes of ring-enhancing lesions:

- Brain abscess
- Tuberculosis
- Primary cerebral neoplasm
- Radiation necrosis
- Toxoplasmosis
- Haemorrhage

Primary tumours commonly causing haemorrhage within the cerebral metastases are:

- Bronchogenic carcinoma (commonest)
- Malignant melanoma

- Choriocarcinoma
- Renal cell carcinoma

3.25 B
3.26 A

Intracranial tumours

Primary brain tumours constitute 50% of all intracranial tumours. More than 70% are supratentorial. Gliomas are commonest followed by meningiomas, schwannomas and others. There is increasing incidence of primary CNS lymphoma as the prevalence of HIV is rising. Acoustic neuroma and meningioma are the most common posterior fossa tumours.

Risk factors

- Brain irradiation
- HIV–CNS lymphoma
- Conditions like tuberous sclerosis and neurofibromatosis

Astrocytoma

These are the most common primary CNS tumours. They represent two ends of the spectrum – on the one end, low-grade gliomas are more common in those in the younger age group, and subependymal giant cell astrocytoma carries the best prognosis; on the other end of spectrum high-grade gliomas (glioblastoma multiforme) are commoner in the elderly and carry a poor prognosis. Oligodendrogliomas have a benign course. They are less infiltrating than astrocytomas and better surgical excision may be possible.

Ependymomas

These tumours are located in the spinal canal and arise from the filum terminale of the spinal cord. They metastasize via CSF. The prognosis is good as total surgical excision is possible.

Primary CNS lymphoma

This occurs independent of systemic lymphoma and is seen in the neuraxis. They are high-grade B-cell tumours, occur commonly in immunocompromised individuals and are associated with Epstein–Barr viral infection. The prognosis is poor compared to systemic lymphoma. They may show marked improvement with steroid therapy, only to recur again quickly. Secondary CNS lymphoma is a manifestation of systemic lymphoma.

Clinical features

The usual symptoms are headache, nausea and vomiting (especially in the morning), confusion, epileptic seizures, visual field defects and focal weakness. In older patients, new-onset headache should be viewed with suspicion. There may be altered mental changes, papilloedema and cranial nerve palsies. In posterior fossa tumours, vertigo, deafness and tinnitus may feature.

Radiology

- *Low-grade astrocytoma*: They may appear isodense or hypodense on CT and calcification may be seen in some. On MRI, they may appear hypointense on T1 and hyperintense on T2, respectively. There is usually no surrounding oedema and they may be confused with cerebral infarct.
- *Anaplastic astrocytoma*: there is contrast enhancement and surrounding oedema.
- *Glioblastoma multiforme*: contrast enhancement and oedema are more marked and they are of heterogeneous intensity. There is a central area of hypointensity due to tumour necrosis and an irregular surrounding, enhancing area. The radiographic changes are non-specific and biopsy is required for diagnosis.
- *Lymphomas*: a solitary, well-defined, rounded mass is seen. On non-contrast CT it appears as hyperdense. There is marked contrast enhancement, but the findings may not be the same in the immunocompromised patient; multiple deposits and ring enhancement are seen.

Differential diagnosis

- Subdural haematoma
- Stroke
- Encephalitis
- Tuberculosis
- Intracerebral haemorrhage
- Brain metastases

Treatment
This depends on the type of the tumour. Supportive treatment in the form of dexamethasone is helpful for cerebral oedema and anticonvulsants like phenytoin are needed if there are seizures. A multidisciplinary team approach including input from neurosurgeons, radiologists and oncologists is essential to decide the best management option.

3.27 B
3.28 A
3.29 B

Meningioma

Meningiomas constitute 15% of all intracranial tumours and 90% are supratentorial. They are benign tumours derived from arachnoid cell rests. They are attached to dura but may invade the skull. The peak incidence is in middle age and they are more common in women.

The common sites are: along the sagittal sinus and over cerebral convexity, cerebellopontine angle and dorsum of the spinal cord.

Clinical features
They may be discovered incidentally on CT or MRI. They are slow growing and symptoms and signs depend on the site of the tumour. They may cause headache, focal weakness, mental changes, seizures and dysphasia.

They may occur as a complication of chemotherapy for cancers like lymphomas.

Some clinical features may be indicative of the location of the meningioma:

- *Olfactory groove*: anosmia
- *Parasagittal*: monoparesis of the contralateral leg
- *Cerebellopontine angle*: vertigo, sensory loss over face, deafness, tinnitus
- *Subfrontal*: mental changes, urinary incontinence
- *Sphenoid ridge*: multiple cranial nerve palsies
- *Intraventricular*: obstructive hydrocephalus

Kennedy–Foster syndrome: olfactory groove meningioma leading to anosmia, ipsilateral optic atrophy and contralateral papilloedema.

Parasagittal meningioma: in parasagittal meningioma, psychosis and parkinsonian features may be seen in addition to other neurological symptoms. It may involve the sagittal sinus and adjacent dural convexity and falx.

Radiology

On CT the lesions appear spherical and well circumscribed. Most of them are hyperdense and enhance uniformly. Hyperostosis of the adjacent bone is usually seen and indicates tumour attachment to the meninges. Enlargement of the arterial and venous grooves indicates enhanced blood supply to the tumour. A 'dural tail' that enhances with the contrast may be seen but is not pathognomonic as it can be seen with some other tumours. Vasogenic oedema is uncommon in supratentorial tumours.

On contrast-enhanced MRI, they enhance intensely and homogeneously but may appear isodense with cerebral cortex on T1- and T2-weighted images.

In parasagittal tumour it is important to know if the tumour has compressed or invaded the superior sagittal sinus as the surgical approach is different.

Some neurosurgeons prefer angiography to determine vascularization and involvement of the venous sinuses. It may also be necessary if pre-operative embolization is planned.

Differential diagnosis

- Gliomas
- Cavernous sinus syndrome
- Primary CNS lymphoma
- Glioblastoma multiforme
- Craniopharyngioma

Treatment

- Supportive treatment in the form of steroids and anticonvulsants may be required.
- Radiotherapy may be used as an adjunct in recurrent or high-grade tumours.

- Radiosurgery helps with tumour control and also for small residual or recurrent tumours.
- Surgery usually gives good results and may be curative.

3.30 B
3.31 D

Cerebellar haemorrhage

Cerebellar haemorrhage is a less common cause of intracranial haemorrhage and results from similar causes as intracerebral haemorrhage (also see section 3.2), for example: hypertension, bleeding diathesis, arteriovenous malformation, cocaine abuse and amyloid angiopathy. Brainstem compression is the most feared complication.

Clinical features
Altered level of consciousness is unusual at presentation. The symptoms may be occipital headache, ataxia, vomiting, dizziness, dysarthria or dysphagia and the symptoms develop over several hours. There may be conjugate lateral gaze palsy towards the side of the haemorrhage or ipsilateral 6th nerve palsy. Later, the patient becomes stuporous or comatose, which may be due to obstructive hydrocephalus or due to brainstem compression; hence haematoma evacuation is essential for survival.

Diagnosis
All patients should have a full blood count, U&E, glucose, lipids, coagulation screen and an ECG. An urgent CT scan of the head should be obtained.

Radiology
The CT scan shows an area of increased density in the posterior fossa. Particular attention is given to any signs of brainstem compression, size and location of the haematoma. Any obstructive hydrocephalus, if present, could be visible. MRI may be required later for further evaluation.

Differential diagnosis

- Subarachnoid haemorrhage
- Subdural haematoma
- Central pontine myelinolysis
- Vestibular neuronitis
- Brainstem syndromes
- Posterior cerebral artery stroke

Treatment
Good, supportive care is very important with attention to the airway and circulation. Patients should be monitored for any signs of raised intracranial pressure.

Surgical evacuation is the treatment except for very small and laterally located haematomas with no signs of clinical deterioration and no evidence of hydrocephalus. A ventricular shunt may be required for hydrocephalus.

3.32 C
3.33 B

Spinal cord compression

Spinal cord compression is a medical emergency and may cause deleterious effects if it is not diagnosed and treated early. The clinical features can be variable and depend on the underlying cause and rate of its development. The symptoms may develop over a few minutes or a few hours in the case of injury, infection or bleeding, or it may be over months in the case of a slow-growing tumour.

Causes

1. *Neoplasms*:
   A. *Intramedullary*: ependymoma, glioma, haemangioblastoma
   B. *Extramedullary*: meningioma, neurofibroma
   C. *Extradural*: metastases from bronchus, breast or prostate
2. *Infections*: tuberculosis, epidural abscess
3. *Trauma*: rupture or disc herniation
4. *Vascular*: epidural haemorrhage, arteriovenous malformation
5. *Miscellaneous*: osteoporotic fracture, Paget's disease, aneurysmal bone cyst, vertebral angioma, multiple myeloma.

Location

- Thoracic spine (70%)
- Lumbosacral spine (20%): mainly from prostate and ovaries
- Cervical spine (10%)

Clinical features

The most common initial symptom is localized pain, which is exacerbated by movement, coughing or sneezing and may worsen when the patient lies flat. There may be numbness and other sensory symptoms in the limbs with loss of sensory modalities like vibration, joint position and pin-prick sensation, the upper limit of which is one or two vertebrae below the site of compression. There may be motor weakness, increased spasticity and deep tendon reflexes may be brisk. Plantar reflex may be extensor and this denotes significant compression. There may be sphincter disturbances in the form of bladder disturbances and bowel dysfunction. The motor and sensory symptoms precede the sphincter involvement. There may be autonomic disturbance in the form of reduced perineal sensation, bladder distension and reduced anal tone and these denote a bad prognosis. Localized vertebral tenderness may signify metastases or infection. With extramedullary lesions, there may be radicular pain, spastic weakness in the legs and sensory loss over the sacral area. With intramedullary lesions there is sacral sparing and a poorly localized burning pain may be present.

Special patterns

- Compression at cervical cord (C4–C5) may lead to quadriplegia and sometimes there may be associated Horner syndrome.

- Compression at thoracic level may present with weakness of legs and sphincter disturbances.
- *Cauda equina syndrome*: there may be radicular pain associated with weakness and sensory loss that may be asymmetrical, reflexes may be diminished and usually there is no sphincter disturbance.
- *Conus medullary syndrome*: sphincter disturbance is prominent here and there may be erectile dysfunction and saddle anaesthesia. The anal and bulbocavernosus reflexes are absent.
- *Brown-Sequard syndrome*: there is ipsilateral weakness and loss of position and joint position sense with loss of pain and temperature on the contralateral side that is one or two levels below the lesion.

Diagnosis
The initial investigations should be directed towards making a diagnosis of cord compression and to find the underlying cause. In the baseline blood tests, inflammatory markers and cancer marker studies should be included. Plain radiographs of the spine should be obtained. The investigation of choice is MRI.

Radiology
Plain X-rays of the spine may show a vertebral collapse or a metastatic lesion. MRI is very helpful in assessing the spinal lesion and the surrounding soft tissue, and it can distinguish between abscess, spinal neoplasm or metastases. MRI of the whole spine should be obtained as multiple metastases may be present. When the disc space is involved the aetiology is most likely to be an infection. In neoplastic lesions, the intervertebral disc is not involved. In case of infection, on T1-weighted images reduced signal intensity is seen associated with peripheral enhancement with gadolinium. In case of vertebral metastases, the lesions appear hypointense on T1-weighted images, which enhance to become isodense with the normal bone marrow.

Treatment
Spinal cord compression is an emergency and treatment is likely to help most people who have not lost sphincter control and who are ambulatory. In cord compression due to malignancy radiotherapy may be required. If the condition is suspected, dexamethasone should be started immediately. The treatment is largely dictated by the underlying aetiology. Surgical decompression through an anterior approach is carried out in infections, disc diseases and tumours as they produce anterior compression.

3.34 D
3.35 A
3.36 A

Brain abscess

Brain abscess is a suppurative collection in brain parenchyma and it is encapsulated. In the initial stages, when no capsule is present, it is called 'cerebritis'. It is fairly uncommon except in some predisposing conditions and in the immunocompromised. The infection can also develop in susceptible individuals in the presence of ischaemia or hypoxia.

The host defence mechanisms and presence of predisposing factors determine the type of infecting organism. The usual infective agents are *Staphylococcus aureus*, streptococci, *Bacteroides* spp, fusobacterium spp, *Pseudomonas aeruginosa*. The uncommon organisms are *H. influenzae*, *N. meningitides* and *Nocardia*. In immunocompromised individuals, *Toxoplasma gondii*, *Cl. neoformans*, *Aspergillus*, *Nocardia* etc.

Risk factors

- Otogenic infections like mastoiditis, otitis media, sinusitis
- Neurosurgical or dental procedures
- Haematogenous spread (25%) from other primary foci like infective endocarditis, lung abscess, bronchiectasis
- Trauma
- Immunodeficiency states
- Cryptogenic (25%)

Usually the location of the abscess is determined by the underlying aetiological factor:

- *Spread from otogenic infection*: temporal lobe or cerebellum.
- *Haematogenous spread*: usually in the MCA territory and often located at grey and white matter junction. The abscesses may be multiple and poorly encapsulated.
- Following dental procedures and from paranasal sinuses: frontal lobes.

Clinical features

The classical triad is fever, headache and focal neurological defects but this is not always present. In fact, fever is present in only 50% of cases. Altered mental status and seizures may be present and in the absence of fever, the features may be those of raised intracranial pressure. The signs and symptoms also depend on the location of the abscess, the virulence of the infecting organism and the intracranial pressure. Neck stiffness is usually not seen except when meninges are involved after rupture of the abscess.

Diagnosis

A thorough history, blood tests including full blood count, CRP, blood glucose, U&E and blood cultures should be carried out. Lumbar puncture should be avoided because of the risk of brain herniation and CSF examination does not add any more information. A CXR must be obtained. A CT or MRI should be arranged urgently.

Radiology

On CT, ring enhancement with a non-enhanced centre, which is due to necrotic tissue with surrounding oedema, is seen. In initial stages when there is cerebritis, no capsule is seen and it may enhance even in the centre. With mature abscess the centre is not enhanced. The margins of the abscess wall are less well enhanced towards the ventricular side than towards the cortex. On non-enhanced CT, the capsule of the abscess may be of reduced attenuation but in cerebral tumours it can be dense, which may be a differentiating feature.

MRI is more sensitive in detecting abscesses than CT. On MRI, enhancement of the capsule occurs with gadolinium. In HIV patients or in the case of haematogenous spread multiple abscesses may be seen.

Differential diagnosis

- Glioblastoma
- Neurocysticercosis
- Tuberculoma
- Haemorrhage
- Metastases

Treatment
High-dose intravenous antibiotics are required for at least 6–8 weeks depending on the infecting organism. Advice from the microbiologists should be sought early. Drainage of abscess is required and can be done by stereotactic approach. Seizures should be controlled with anticonvulsants. Resolution of the abscess should be ascertained by repeating a CT of the head or MRI.

Section 4: Cardiovascular System

Questions

4.1   A 60-year-old woman presents with dyspnoea of 3 days' duration, is feeling light-headed and her blood pressure is low, at 90/50 mmHg. She is known to have end-stage renal disease and is on dialysis. Her CXR and CT are shown. What is the most likely diagnosis?

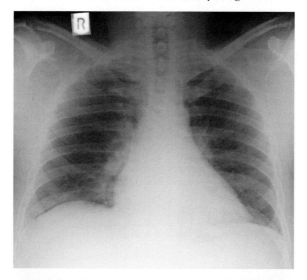

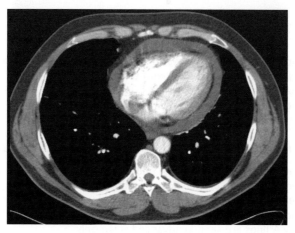

A. CCF
B. Cardiac tamponade
C. Constrictive pericarditis
D. Pulmonary embolism

4.2   All the following are true of cardiac tamponade except:

    A. Kussmaul's sign is very uncommon.
    B. Echocardiography is the investigation of choice.
    C. MRI is the investigation of choice.
    D. Pulsus paradoxus is a characteristic feature of tamponade.

4.3   A 64-year-old man presented with dyspnoea that developed over a few hours. He is known to have ischaemic heart disease. A CXR was arranged (shown) and pulmonary oedema is suspected. Please choose the correct statement:

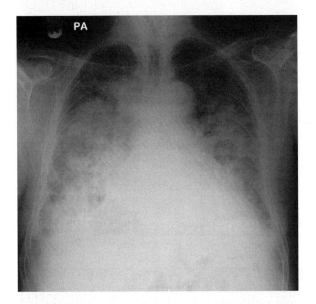

    A. Pulmonary oedema is always secondary to underlying cardiac diseases.
    B. The signs on CXR correlate with the PCWP.
    C. Dobutamine is contraindicated.
    D. Pulmonary oedema is always symmetrical.

4.4   All the following are true regarding pulmonary oedema except:

    A. Kerley B lines are seen only in pulmonary oedema.
    B. Kerley B lines run perpendicular to the pleural surface.
    C. Upper-lobe diversion of the pulmonary blood flow is indicative of early pulmonary venous hypertension.
    D. Kerley A lines are seen in advanced stage only.

4.5 A 40-year-old tall and thin man presented with complaints of severe chest pain and shortness of breath. His past medical history consisted of aspiration of a pneumothorax 1 year ago. A CXR and a CT were carried out and are shown. What is the most likely diagnosis?

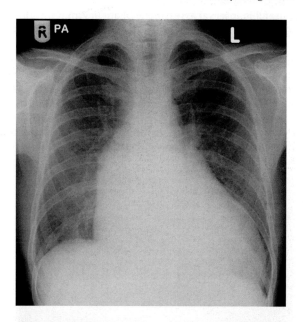

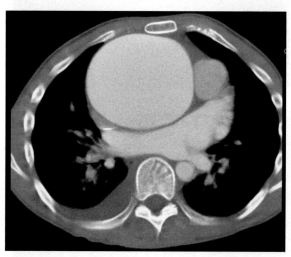

A. Pneumothorax
B. Dilatation of the aorta
C. Pericardial tamponade
D. Mediastinal mass

4.6   All the following are true except:

   A. Aortography is the investigation of choice for diagnosis.
   B. Long-term beta-blockers should be considered for patients with dilatation of the aorta.
   C. MRI is useful in interval assessment of aneurysm.
   D. Aortography may not define the true diameter of the dilatation.

4.7   A 72-year-old man was brought to the A&E department with a history of abdominal pain radiating to the back. He had been feeling light-headed and collapsed at home without loss of consciousness. His feet were cold and he was hypotensive. His blood tests showed leucocytosis and mildly raised urea and creatinine. A CT scan of the abdomen was carried out and is shown. What is the most likely diagnosis?

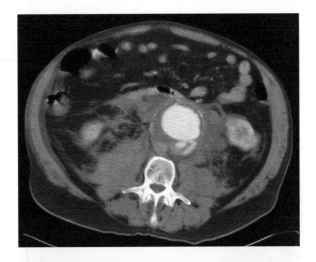

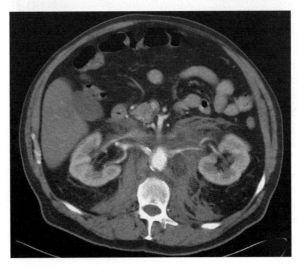

A. Acute pancreatitis
B. Perforated bowel
C. Dilated abdominal aorta
D. Rupture of abdominal aorta

4.8 Please choose the correct statement:

A. Aortic aneurysm is more common in women.
B. Most of the aneurysms are below the renal arteries.
C. Most of the aneurysms are above the renal arteries.
D. Ultrasound with Doppler flow is almost always diagnostic of rupture of the abdominal aneurysm.

4.9 A 58-year-old man presented with symptoms of dyspnoea and chest pain. His past medical history consisted of coronary artery disease and an MI 1 year previously. A CXR was carried out and is shown. What is the diagnosis?

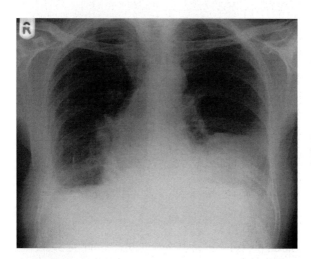

A. Left ventricular aneurysm
B. Left atrial enlargement
C. Dilated cardiomyopathy
D. Round pneumonia

4.10 What should be the treatment in this case?

A. Regular monitoring
B. Optimize his angina and heart failure drugs
C. Surgical treatment
D. Antibiotics

4.11 Choose the correct statement:

    A. True left ventricular aneurysms are very prone to rupture.

    B. False left ventricular aneurysms are very prone to rupture.

    C. Excision of the true ventricular aneurysm should be done even in asymptomatic patients.

    D. True left ventricular aneurysm is seen exclusively as a complication of MI.

4.12 A 35-year-old patient presented with complaints of fatigue, headache and pain in legs on walking. There was also a history of chest pains. In the context of this history and the image shown, please choose the correct answer:

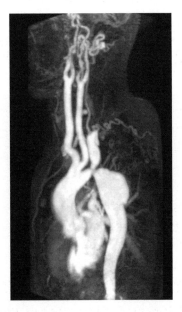

    A. The blood pressure in the lower limbs would be expected to be higher than upper limbs.

    B. Subarachnoid haemorrhage may be a complication.

    C. The condition is more common in females.

    D. The condition affects the aorta proximal to the origin of the left subclavian artery.

4.13 All the following are correct in relation to coarctation of the aorta except:

    A. The '3 sign' when seen is pathognomonic.

    B. Rib-notching is usually symmetrical.

    C. Rib-notching is seen only in coarctation of the aorta.

    D. Echocardiography is diagnostic.

Answers

4.1 B
4.2 C

Cardiac tamponade

Cardiac tamponade is a medical emergency and can be fatal if not diagnosed and treated early. Normally there is small amount of fluid (15–50 ml) between visceral and parietal pericardium. If the volume of fluid increases it may be significant enough to cause a rise in pressure within the pericardial cavity and impair ventricular filling and consequently cause cardiac tamponade. The rate at which the fluid develops is important. If it is a slow process up to 1–2 L may be present by the time the patients become symptomatic but if it occurs quickly or the pericardium is stiff then it may compromise the circulation even with smaller volumes.

Causes
Pericarditis due to any cause can lead to tamponade. Some common aetiological factors are mentioned below:

- Malignancy
- Uraemia
- Idiopathic
- Trauma and cardiac surgery
- Infections like tuberculosis, viral, HIV
- Anticoagulants (haemopericardium)

Clinical features
Signs and symptoms are due to reduced cardiac output and increased intracardiac pressures. The patients are hypotensive and dyspnoeic on exertion or also at rest. The JVP is raised and heart sounds are diminished. An important clinical finding is pulsus paradoxus, i.e. fall of systolic pressure by 10 mmHg on inspiration. These findings are usually seen in acute cardiac tamponade but when it develops slowly, the signs and symptoms may be that of CCF. Kussmaul's sign may be positive but is a very uncommon finding.

Diagnosis
Baseline blood tests should be carried out and also ESR, ANCA and rheumatoid factor. On ECG sinus tachycardia or conduction disturbances are seen. The QRS complexes may be of low voltage and electrical alternans may be seen. A CXR should be obtained. Echocardiography is the investigation of choice.

Radiology
The CXR may show an enlarged globular heart or it may appear bottle shaped. In acute tamponade the heart size may appear to be normal. When the heart size is increased but the pulmonary vasculature is not prominent tamponade should be suspected.

CT or MRI may be helpful when echocardiography is inconclusive in a small number of patients. They may also help to detect any causative factors like haemorrhage, tuberculosis and malignant process.

Treatment
Cardiac tamponade is a medical emergency. The pericardiocentesis should be performed under echocardiograpic guidance. Full resuscitation facilities should be available. The other option is to do limited thoracotomy. Treatment of the underlying condition should be considered.

4.3 B
4.4 A

Pulmonary oedema

Pulmonary oedema occurs due to extravasation of fluid from the pulmonary vasculature into the lung interstitium and eventually into alveolar space, and is due to disturbance in the haemodynamics between the hydrostatic and oncotic pressures, disruption of the alveolar-capillary membrane or due to lymphatic obstruction. In some conditions the exact mechanism is not clear. It can be divided into cardiogenic and non-cardiogenic types.

Causes

1. *Cardiogenic*:
   - Valvular heart disease: mitral stenosis, decompensated aortic valve disease and mitral regurgitation
   - Acute myocardial infarction
   - Cardiomyopathies, e.g. hypertrophic, ischaemic
   - Left ventricular thrombus
   - Left atrial myxoma
2. *Non-cardiogenic*:
   - Hypoalbuminaemia
   - High altitudes
   - Narcotic overdose
   - ARDS
   - Neurogenic
   - Re-expansion pulmonary oedema following rapid aspiration of pneumothorax
   - Left atrial myxoma

Clinical features
The main symptom is dyspnoea along with signs of sympathetic stimulation. The patients may be very breathless, even at rest, and they may appear very anxious and clammy. They may have a cough with pink and frothy sputum, which is usually seen in very advanced stages. On physical examination, there is tachycardia and tachypnoea. There are bibasilar crepitations and a third heart sound may be heard. The BP is usually elevated.

Diagnosis
The baseline blood tests should be carried out along with cardiac markers like CK and troponin I. The ABGs may show hypoxaemia. ECG may show

tachycardia and signs of acute MI if that is the underlying cause. An urgent CXR should be obtained. An echocardiography with Doppler flow helps distinguish between cardiogenic and non-cardiogenic pulmonary oedema and can also identify valvular heart lesions. Measurement of PCWP also helps to differentiate between cardiogenic and non-cardiogenic causes.

Radiology

The CXR is helpful in differentiating pulmonary oedema from other causes of dyspnoea. It can also help determine the severity of the pulmonary oedema. The CXR findings may correlate with the PCWP.

In a normal CXR the right descending pulmonary trunk is the most prominent vascular structure. In early stages it becomes less prominent and instead the blood vessels in the upper lobe become more prominent. This is a pointer of pulmonary venous hypertension.

In moderate cases, the Kerley B lines are seen. Small pleural effusion may be noted and also interstitial pulmonary oedema. This is seen in the form of areas of opacity or reticular shadowing and peribronchial thickening. The Kerley B lines are seen due to accumulation of fluid in the interlobular septa and in their contained lymphatics. They are usually seen near the costophrenic angle and appear perpendicular to the pleural surface. In a sudden onset of pulmonary oedema or in severe cases similar lines may be seen in the central portion of the lung, called 'Kerley A lines'. Kerley B lines are seen in some other conditions as well.

In severe cases, an alveolar-filling pattern is seen. The opacities are usually perihilar or in the basal lung areas. Sometimes they may be asymmetrical, which may be due to underlying lung disease. Cardiomegaly or left atrial enlargement may be seen.

Treatment

The aim is to improve oxygenation and ventilation and reduction of preload and systemic vascular resistance (afterload):

- Oxygen therapy should be begun immediately. Non-invasive ventilation should be considered early. Mechanical ventilation may be required if oxygenation is not improving or in the presence of haemodynamic compromise.
- Morphine controls the pain and also the signs of sympathetic stimulation.
- Pharmacological agents that help reduce preload are: loop diuretics, nitrates, morphine and ACE-inhibitors.
- Inotropic agents like dopamine and dobutamine help improve myocardial contractility and in the presence of severe LV dysfunction.

Causes of Kerley B lines (other than pulmonary oedema):

- Lymphangitis carcinomatosis
- Lymphangioleiomyomatosis
- Lymphatic obstruction secondary to tumour or irradiation
- Pneumoconiosis

Causes of asymmetrical pulmonary oedema:

- Gravitational
- COPD

- Pulmonary atresia
- Pulmonary embolism (contralateral side)
- In presence of mediastinal tumours
- Left atrial thrombus
- Re-expansion of lung after aspiration of pneumothorax

4.5 B
4.6 A

Aortic root dilatation

Aortic root dilatation (ARD) is associated with a wide range of clinical entities. It can be divided into a true dilatation and a false type. In true dilatation all three layers of aortic wall are involved but in the false type the intima and media are disrupted and the dilatation is lined by the adventitial layer. It is a progressive disease and grows at the rate of 0.1–0.4 cm/year.

Causes

1. Atherosclerosis
2. Congenital:
   - Bicuspid aortic valve
3. Connective tissue disorders:
   - Marfan's syndrome (cystic medial necrosis)
   - Ehler–Danlos syndrome
4. Infection:
   - Syphilitic
   - Tuberculosis
   - Mycotic aneurysm
5. Inflammatory and degenerative:
   - Giant cell arteritis
   - Takayasu's arteritis
   - Rheumatoid
6. Trauma

Clinical features
ARD may present with chest pain, shortness of breath or cough. Pressure on the adjacent structures may cause dysphagia and hoarseness of voice. The aneurysm of the ascending aorta may present with symptoms of heart failure. The most feared complication is rupture, which can be life threatening.

Diagnosis
Often the diagnosis is made incidentally, when a CXR is carried out for some other reason. The baseline bloods and ECG should be obtained. An echocardiogram is helpful in defining size of the aorta and also to identify valvular lesions. Transoesophageal echocardiography is superior to transthoracic echocardiography. The CT scan and MRI are important diagnostic tools.

Radiology

- The CXR shows a widened mediastinum and may also show displacement of the trachea or the left main bronchus.

- Aortography is commonly carried out preoperatively and helps to find the extent of the aneurysm and the involvement of its branches. The true size of the dilatation may not be defined and dissection may be missed. There is also a small risk of stroke from a laminated thrombus.
- *CT scan*: The CT is a very useful diagnostic test. It can help define the size and extent of dilatation, the involvement of the branch vessels and also presence of dissection, rupture or intramural thrombus.
- With MRI and MR angiography the advantage is that it does not involve radiation or nephrotoxic contrast infusion. It provides very precise assessment of the extent of the dilatation, involvement of the branch vessels and the relationship to the surrounding structures. It also detects regurgitation and fistulae. MRI is a very useful tool for the interval assessment of the dilatation.

Treatment

- The patients who have evidence of dilatation should receive beta-blockers on a long-term basis and high blood pressure should be controlled. This is particularly important in Marfan's syndrome, with evidence of aortic root dilatation. These patients are at increased risk of dissection or rupture when the diameter of dilatation is > 6 cm.
- Surgery is considered once the size of the dilatation is > 6 cm or it has grown at a rate of more than 1 cm/year. But in case of Marfan's syndrome surgery should be considered once the dilatation is > 5 cm.

4.7 D
4.8 B

Ruptured abdominal aortic aneurysm

Ruptured abdominal aortic aneurysm (AAA) occurs when the dilated aorta continues to expand. This is a life-threatening condition and is fatal unless urgent repair is carried out. They are more frequent in males. In most cases the aneurysm is seen below the renal arteries and is usually due to atherosclerosis. The prognosis depends on the size of the AAA and is also associated with coronary artery or cerebrovascular disease.

Risk factors

- Male sex
- Smoking
- Advanced age
- Hypertension
- COPD (low FEV1)
- Family history

Clinical features
The AAA may be asymptomatic but pain may occur if they continue to expand. When severe pain occurs in the presence of a palpable aorta, rupture must be excluded urgently. There may be a history of back pain and syncope. Sometimes the rupture can occur without any warning symptoms.

Hypotension may be present and there may be a tender mass palpable in the abdomen.

The following may be associated with increased mortality:

- Systolic hypotension of < 80 mmHg
- Respiratory failure
- Renal impairment
- Cardiac arrest
- History of loss of consciousness

Diagnosis
Baseline blood tests should be carried out and blood grouped and cross-matched. The AXR usually shows calcification but may not be seen in 25% of cases. An ultrasound of the abdomen with Doppler flow should be obtained. A CT or MRI is more definitive for diagnosis.

Radiology
The ultrasound shows the presence of the aneurysm and can also detect the mural thrombus but it may fail to show the leakage. It has other limitations like overlying bowel gas and obesity. Hence, if rupture is suspected a CT or MRI should be arranged.

The CT is an excellent test and is usually diagnostic. It shows the presence of dilatation, intramural thrombus and the site of the rupture. The branch vessels and the surrounding structures can be evaluated, including the kidneys. The downside is that it involves contrast injection.

MRI is also a valuable tool and it can be helpful if contrast injection has to be avoided as in presence of renal failure.

Differential diagnosis

- Perforated bowel
- Acute cholecystitis
- Pancreatitis
- Renal colic
- Bowel ischaemia

Treatment
The initial aim is to stabilize the patient and attention should be paid to the airway, breathing and circulation. The definitive treatment is surgery, which consists of repair of the rupture with a prosthetic graft.

4.9 A
4.10 C
4.11 B

Left ventricular aneurysm

Left ventricular aneurysm (LVA) is a thin-walled bulge through a weak area of the left ventricle. It is a complication of myocardial infarction.

It is of two types:

- *True LVA*: it is usually a complication of large anteroseptal MI. There may be dilatation of the left ventricle and the regional wall movement may be abnormal. Rupture is uncommon as the aneurysmal ventricular wall is replaced by fibrous tissue. *Causes*: MI, Chagas' disease, trauma, sarcoidosis, congenital (rare).
- *False LVA*: it occurs after trauma or MI and at abnormal locations on the ventricular wall. They are prone to complications like rupture and surgical treatment should be considered early. *Causes*: MI, post-cardiac surgery and septic pericarditis.

Clinical features
These include angina and dyspnoea; palpitations due to arrhythmias are not unusual. Systemic thromboembolism can cause stroke or limb ischaemia. Heart failure due to paradoxical filling of the aneurysm during systole may be seen. Syncope and sudden death can also occur.

Diagnosis
The ECG shows persistent Q-waves and anterior ST elevation. A CXR should be arranged, which may show the aneurysm or cardiac enlargement but is not reliable. Two-dimensional echocardiography is a sensitive test but left ventriculography is considered to be the gold standard. Echo-cardiography helps to differentiate true from false LVA and it can detect intramural thrombus. MRI very accurately shows LVA and left ventricular volume. It can also show intramural thrombus.

Differential diagnosis

- Cardiomyopathy
- Round pneumonia
- Lung cancer
- Solitary pulmonary nodule

Treatment
The definitive treatment is surgical. Medical treatment may help control symptoms. Asymptomatic patients do not require treatment. Surgical treatment is indicated in the presence of symptoms of heart failure, arrhythmias and angina. It is also indicated in false LVA and in congenital aneurysms.

4.12 A
4.13 C

Coarctation of the aorta

Coarctation of the aorta (CoA) is a congenital narrowing of the aorta and is seen commonly distal to the origin of the left subclavian artery though it can occur anywhere along the length of the aorta. It is more common in males. An important characteristic is development of collateral circulation around the obstruction.

Clinical features
It may be asymptomatic and the condition is detected when a murmur or

hypertension are found incidentally. The patients may have headaches, fatigue, chest pain, cold peripheries and claudication or weakness in the legs. The upper limbs and thorax may be better developed as compared to the lower limbs. On examination, there may be a delay in the pulses in the lower limb as compared to the upper limb and a difference in the blood pressure. A mid-systolic murmur is heard anteriorly or may be heard over the spinous process.

Diagnosis
A CXR may be normal or may show rib-notching. It is bilateral and seen mainly affecting ribs 3–9. Rib-notching is seen only in longstanding CoA and it should be remembered that it is not specific to CoA. It may show the '3 sign', which is due to indentation of the aorta at the site of coarctation with pre- and post-stenotic dilatation; if this is present, it is pathognomonic.

A two-dimensional (2D) echocardiography helps with diagnosis and shows the site and extent of the coarctation. With Doppler, the pressure gradient across the narrowing can be made. MRI is a very sensitive test but is not commonly used as a diagnostic tool. It provides useful information on the site and extent of the obstruction and the state of the collateral vessels. It can be useful for follow up. Angiography with selective ventriculography and aortography, though not used routinely, may give additional information in the presence of other anomalies.

Treatment
The definitive treatment is surgical; resection and end-to-end anastomoses or a subclavian flap procedure is usually carried out. Medical treatment in the form of diuretics may be required when symptoms of heart failure are present. Hypertension should be treated if present.

Associations of CoA

- Turner's syndrome
- Bicuspid aortic valve
- Ventricular septal defect
- Subarachnoid haemorrhage due to Berry aneurysms of the circle of Willis.

Other causes of rib-notching

- Aortic thrombosis
- Takayasu's arteritis
- Pulmonary artery atresia
- Tetralogy of Fallot
- Blalock–Taussig shunt

Section 5: Musculoskeletal System

Questions

5.1 A 75-year-old woman presented with pain in her legs, mobility problems, headaches and deafness. An X-ray was carried out and is shown. What is the likely diagnosis?

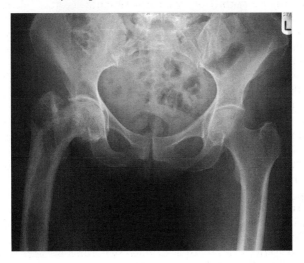

A. Fibrous dysplasia
B. Paget's disease
C. Metastatic lesion
D. Osteoarthritis

5.2 All the following are true of Paget's disease except:

A. Very high ALP levels may be indicative of skull involvement.
B. Sarcoma is a rare complication of Paget's disease.
C. Serum calcium levels are always elevated.
D. Serum total ALP can be used to assess the response to treatment.

5.3 A 20-year-old man had presented with a history of pain, which increased on knee movement, and swelling. His blood tests showed a slightly raised white cell count and a raised ALP. A knee X-ray was carried out and is shown. What is the most likely diagnosis?

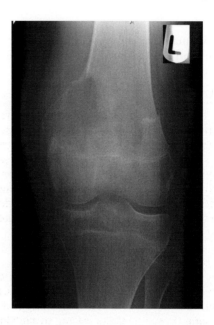

A. Osteosarcoma
B. Osteomyelitis
C. Ewing's sarcoma
D. Haematoma

5.4 All the following are true regarding the above diagnosis except:

A. Presence of the Codman triangle on the X-ray of the affected area is not specific to osteosarcoma.
B. A very raised ALP may be indicative of lung metastases.
C. Response to neoadjuvant chemotherapy is a prognostic marker.
D. Pathological fractures are extremely common.

Section 5: Musculoskeletal System

Answers

5.1 A
5.2 D

Paget's disease

Paget's disease of the bone is a condition of bone remodelling. Excessive bone resorption due to increased activity of osteoclasts causes osteoblastic new bone formation. It may affect various areas of the skeleton. The new bone formed is structurally abnormal and hence may lead to deformities and fractures. It may also lead to local complications secondary to bone expansion. There is a tendency to affect the axial skeleton, long bones and skull, but virtually any bone in the body may be affected. The disease can be divided into the following three phases: lytic phase, intermediate or mixed phase and sclerotic phase.

Clinical features
Patients may be symptomatic and may be diagnosed incidentally when being investigated for other conditions. Amongst symptoms, pain is the most frequent complaint. There may be a bony deformity and this may be seen as bowing of the bone (femur or tibia), leading to mobility problems; furthermore when areas adjacent to joints are involved there may be secondary osteoarthritis. There may also be spinal deformities, compression fracture and spinal canal stenosis. When there is skull involvement there may be dizziness, vertigo, headaches, tinnitus and deafness. Sometimes the presentation may be due to complications of Paget's disease including congestive cardiac failure, fractures and focal weakness due to nerve root involvement. The involved extremity is warm and tender.

Diagnosis
A combination of biochemical findings and radiological abnormalities help with diagnosis. Alkaline phosphatase levels are elevated. Bone-specific isoenzyme should be obtained. Urinary hydroxyproline levels may be elevated. Raised ALP and urinary hydroxyproline levels are biochemical markers for bone formation and resorption. Very high levels of ALP (> 10 times) are seen with skull involvement and one other site involvement. Serum total ALP also helps to assess the response to therapy. Urinary and serum deoxypyridinoline and N-telopeptide and C-telopeptide levels are newer bone resorption markers and their levels should decrease in the urine. Serum calcium and phosphorus levels are within normal limits.

Radiology
The radiographic appearances may show evidence of lysis or new bone formation. Some areas may show sclerotic appearances. Usually a mixture of sclerotic changes and lytic lesions is most commonly seen. In the skull, a cotton wool pattern of increased density is seen. An increased thickness of the ver-

tebral cortex gives a 'picture frame' appearance. In the pelvic bones thickening of the iliopectineal lines and sclerosis gives the 'brim sign'. Sarcomas are a rare complication of Paget's disease. In this situation CT or MRI may be helpful. Radionuclide studies may be helpful in defining the extent of the disease.

Treatment

Medical treatment in the form of bisphosphonates is needed to treat the symptoms and complications of Paget's disease, which include bone pain, deformities, fractures, local compressive complications and joint involvement. NSAIDs can be used for pain. Biochemical markers should be used to monitor disease activity. A ^{99m}Tc bone scan and radiographs also demonstrate increased skeletal structure.

5.3   B
5.4   C

Osteosarcoma

Osteosarcoma is a highly malignant tumour affecting children and young adults in their second or third decades of life (most commonly between the ages of 10 and 20 years) and is the second most common bone tumour. Osteosarcoma in those in the older age group is secondary to a pre-existing condition like Paget's disease or after radiation therapy. It is commoner in males. Its hallmark is production of malignant osteoid.

It affects the metaphyses of long bone. The most common site is around knee or the distal femur, proximal tibia and proximal humerus.

Clinical features

The usual clinical features are pain and swelling in the affected area. The pain is worst with activity. Pathological fractures are not very common. Osteosarcoma may metastasize to lung or bone.

Diagnosis

Along with other baseline tests LDH and ALP should be checked. Patients with a high ALP result are very likely to have lung metastasis.

Radiology

Initially plain films should be obtained of the affected region. A CXR and a CT of the chest should also be carried out. The lesions of the affected area may show osteolytic or osteoblastic features and the characteristic Codman triangle may be seen, which is due to elevation of periosteum at the margin of the soft tissue mass. A spiculated periosteal reaction called 'sunburst appearance' may also be seen. The Codman triangle is not specific to osteosarcoma. MRI is invaluable in surgical staging and to define the extent of the tumour. It may also give information on medullary extension and involvement of an adjacent joint. Angiography may be required to assess the response to chemotherapy.

Differential diagnosis

- Osteomyelitis
- Trauma/haematoma

- Osteoblastoma
- Histiocytosis X
- Ewing's sarcoma

Treatment

Close co-operation between oncologists and orthopaedic surgeons is required. The treatment of osteosarcoma is surgical and definitive resection should be aimed at, with clear bone margins. The recurrence rate has been very high due to micrometastases and hence nowadays neoadjuvant chemotherapy is used, which reduces the size of the tumour and facilitates its removal. Patients who show good response to neoadjuvant chemotherapy have a good prognosis as compared to those who do not.